A DESCRIPTION OF THE

CRIMES AND HORRORS

IN THE INTERIOR OF

WARBURTON'S PRIVATE MAD-HOUSE

AT HOXTON,

COMMONLY CALLED WHITMORE HOUSE:

DEDICATED TO THE

RIGHT HONOURABLE VISCOUNT SIDMOUTH,
LATE SECRETARY OF STATE, &C.

AND THE

RIGHT HONOURABLE LORD REDESDALE,
LATE CHANCELLOR OF IRELAND, &C.

'I can a tale unfold, whose lightest word
'Will harrow up thy soul.'

London
Spradabach Publishing
2023

Spradabach Publishing
BM Box Spradabach
London WC1N 3XX

*A Description of the Crimes and Horrors
in the Interior of Warburton's Mad-House,
At Hoxton, Commonly Called Whitmore House*

First published in 1825

First Spradabach edition published 2023
© Spradabach Publishing 2023

Interior design by Alex Kurtagic

ISBN 978-1-909606-39-5

British Library Cataloguing-in-Publication Data:
A catalogue record for this book is available from the British Library.

DEDICATED

Right Hon. Viscount Sidmouth,
Late Secretary of State, &c.

Right Honourable Lord Redesdale,
Late Lord Chancellor of Ireland, &c.

MY LORDS,

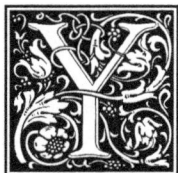

Y ou are egregiously mistaken if you expect this dedication to be couched in the usual style of servile flattery. I am none of the fulsome breed, but a plain downright Englishman, and take you to be the exact sort of fellows fit to be exposed in a Dedication to a Work describing an Establishment of which any honest man would blush to acknowledge himself the patron.

You, my Lord Sidmouth,[1] have a son,[2] to whom, in a state of incurable madness, you gave the Clerkship of the Pells,[3] in Ireland; and for whose imbecility the public are taxed with 3000l. *per annum*, of which Warburton, the mad-house keeper, receives one half-for doing nothing but laugh at your credulity, as you do at that of John Bull.

You, John Mitford, Lord Redesdale,[4] have had a relation, a John Mitford,[5] also in this House, who was protected there to write libels against the Crown and Government, in conjunction with your relation, Viscountess Perceval[6] and her illustrious friend.[7] You paid for Mr. Mitford's protection, to

---

1   Henry Addington, 1st Viscount Sidmouth, PC (1757 – 1844) was not Secretary of State, as says in the title of the dedication, but Prime Minister (1801 - 1804) and later Home Secretary (1812 - 1822). Previously, he had been elected Member of Parliament for Devizes in 1784, become Speaker for the House of Commons of Great Britain in 1800 and of the United Kingdom in 1801.—Ed.

2   Hon. Henry Addington jnr (d. 1823). —Ed.

3   The Pells Office was a department of the Exchequer. All receipts and payments were entered into a roll of parchment called *introitta*, and all moneys issued into another called *exitus*. The Clerk of the Pells was responsible for making a statement of all the moneys issued. The post was abolished in 1834. —Ed.

4   John Freeman-Mitford, 1st Baron Redesdale (1748 - 1830) was Lord Chancellor of Ireland from 1802 till 1806. —Ed.

5   (1782 - 1831). —Ed.

6   Lady Bridget Perceval, daughter-in-law of John James Perceval, 3rd Earl of Egmont (1737/8 - 1822). —Ed.

7   Caroline of Brunswick-Wolfenbüttel (1768 - 1821), the Princes of Wales at the time. —Ed.

Warburton, more than 300l. in nine months, when tried at the bar of the King's Bench, before Lord Ellenborough.[8]

Now, Messrs. Sidmouth and Redesdale, 'read this, and this, and know I know your worthiness.' After Lord Sidmouth's prosecution of the poor Plymouth tinman, and Lord Redesdale's prosecution of the Catholic Priest O'Neil, and his abuse of Dr. Troy and Lord Fingal,[9] I have little hope, you, Messrs. my Lords, will do more than blush for shame after you have read this family work; it is ready at your service, so 'now to dinner with what appetite you may.'

My Lords,
I am a Man whom you do not like,
and
Who neither values your Friendship,
Nor dreads your enmity,
THE PUBLISHER

---

8 For John Mitford's own account, see *The important trial of John Mitford, Esq., on the prosecution of Lady Viscountess Perceval, for perjury at Guildhall, on Thursday, Feb. 24, 1814, before Lord Ellenborough : forming a clue to the discussions which took place relative to the affairs of Her Royal Highness the Princess of Wales, in the beginning of the year 1813 / by the Editor of the News : with an appendix containing a number of original letter from Lady Perceval and John Mitford, Esq., never yet published* (London: T.A. Phipps, 1814). —Ed.

9 Arthur James Plunkett, 8th Earl of Fingall KP (1759 – 1835) was prominent supporter of Catholic emancipation. —Ed.

Table of Contents

Note on This Edition

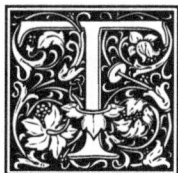

he present text is based on the Benrow edition published in London in 1825. It is reproduced here in its entirety.

The spelling, punctuation, and capitalisation appear as in the original, except (i) blockquotes have been taken out of quotation marks; (ii) commas and periods have been placed outside closing parentheses when appearing just inside; and (iii) quotation marks, which appeared variously as double or single, have been harmonised as single. The italisation also appears as in the original, except the titles of books mentioned in the text have been taken out of quotation marks and italicised, as per modern convention. Typographical errors have been silently corrected.

A complement of editorial footnotes have been added and marked as such.

An index has been generated.

Warburton's Private Mad-House, &c. &c.

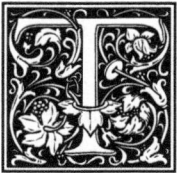

The name of Warburton, called by mistake Doctor, has again become notorious, by his evidence given at the Freemason's Hall, against the Earl Portsmouth,[1] which is of a nature that no one can comprehend. It might almost be inferred from it, that, accustomed to brood over insane person's cases, his own mind had become diseased. He spoke like a madman, endeavouring to persuade his auditors that he was the only one amongst them *compos mentis*; that they must be deranged, because they were unable to comprehend his ravings.

---

1   John Charles Wallop, 3rd Earl of Portsmouth (1767 - 1853). —Ed.

The writer has heard Mr. Warburton make use of the same words he did upon Lord Portsmouth's trial fifty times over, and applied them to as many different cases.

Mr. Warburton is as fond of his 'shades of distinction,' (which, by the bye, he is unable to define) as Ephraim Jenkinson, in *The Vicar of Wakefield*, was of 'the cosmogony, or creation of the world,' and both had an equal knowledge of their subject. What the opinion of Warburton may be now thought of by our doubting Chancellor, we do not know; what he did once think of it, we are well aware. Not many years ago, a fellow of the name of Bowler fired a blunderbuss at a man to whom he bore deadly enmity; he was lodged in gaol, he had a large fortune, and tried every means to escape justice; at last, a jury, with Mr. Warburton at their head, overhauled him in Newgate, and pronounced him insane. The chancellor, the judge, and the jury, disbelieved Mr. Warburton's council, and Bowler was hanged. So much for the value of an opinion which Mr. Warburton gave at Free Mason's Hall, backed by forty years' experience.

Let us now see how Mr. Warburton gained that experience, and the manner he practices in his Inquisition at Hoxton, to cure insane persons. It is a rule in that house, which was always in the mouths of the keepers, particularly an inhuman scoundrel named Jemmy Davis, who had charge of the Hall, and its wretched beings—'If a man comes in here mad, we'll keep him so; if he is in his senses, we'll soon drive him out of them;'—and that they acted up to this infernal motto, I will make as clear as the sun at noon day, before I lay down my pen. I will not mince the matter because Mr. Warburton has immense wealth in his hands, and a phalanx of *materia medica* to support him, (though I am told that his son, Dr. Warburton, of Clifford Street, lately married to the daughter of Dr. Abernethy, is now sole physician to Hoxton, with the assistance of Dunston, the apothecary, Warburton's son-in-law, of whom I have to speak hereafter; as also Mr. Rogers, dismissed for his humanity; Mr. Penlington, an obscure, illiterate, and vulgar nephew of his, who kept a chandler's shop, had moreover the honour of being keeper to our late venerable monarch, whose strait-waistcoats were washed and mended under the care of Mrs. Bruning, the housekeeper, since succeeded by the worthy Mistress Taylor. Of that Windsor job I have much to say, but I shall first begin with the Establishment, and then glance off to its different branches.

If there is in the breasts of men one sacred spark of love, humanity, or pity, it will be called forth for helpless beings, lashed and tortured by fellows deserving of a gibbet; and where, both by men and women, deeds are done that shun the face of day, and enormities practised that cry aloud to heaven for vengeance.

Let us first begin with Mr. Warburton, and then, in regular detail, proceed to his honest servants, such as the brother of orator Hunt, who cleans knives and washes dishes in the kitchen in order to cure him of insanity. And on a careful exposure of this diabolical establishment, I doubt not all will agree with me in opinion, that these 'lawless houses under the law' should be done away with entirely, as a disgrace to human nature. The angel of death moves through them with secret and murderous strides; like Doctor Sangrado's patients, in *Gil Blas*, all that die are wrote down—'cured!'

Thomas Warburton, esq. keeper of the asylums for lunatics, Whitmore House, Hoxton—Mare Street, Hackney—Bethnal Green—and several minor establishments in Kingsland Road, &c. &c., was originally a butcher's-boy in the country, and fled to London before he had served the term of his apprenticeship, for having a bastard-child swore to him. He was first employed under the porter at the gate of Whitmore House, to beat coats, clean shoes, and carry messages, for which he was rewarded with his meat. Being expert at conveying liquor into the house for the keepers to dispose of amongst their patients, (a practice still pursued) he obtained a footing as a servant, and in that situation, by a little help, and much industry, he learned to read and write. His strength of body (a necessary qualification for a demon in one of those hells), and his zeal, raised him to the dignity of a keeper, and he assumed the controul of the lash under happy auspices. He is more than six feet high, broad shoulders, heavy built, with knock-knees, and a visage on which is a proboscis three inches long, quite sufficient to frighten a person of weak mind and delicate nerves into a fit of insanity. I have heard one of the myrmidons who attended at Windsor say, that the old King could not bear to look upon him, and used to exclaim: 'Take away that fellow with the long nose—take him away—away—away.' In time, he attained the confidential office of first keeper (lately held by Tom Harris), and by his treatment of the lunatics under his care, gained the good graces of his mistress, who, upon the death of her husband, married him, and he became ruler over the mansion of affliction. Tom possessed a great deal of low cunning, and insinuating manners, which worked him into the good graces of many not awake to his duplicity. When he was raised to his mistress' bed, there were not many patients in the house, and no regular medical attendant. Tom having scraped together two hundred pounds, presented it to the late Doctor Willis, and engaged him for that sum annually, to recommend his house. He soon had every ward in it filled, and managed to get a lease of the extensive premises at Hoxton for a mere trifle. I have heard how this was done. The keeper of St. Luke's had a son, an apothecary—one of Tom's daughters is that son's wife, and he physics the patients to some purpose.

The visiting physicians are not to blame if they make good reports of Hoxton mad-house, as they are deceived. A week or two before their visitation, the patients are better fed, and more kindly used, Tommy himself sometimes dines with them in the parlour, in order that he may say—'Oh, the patients live so well I frequently dine at their table from choice!' The house is moreover cleaned, and new clothes distributed to those in rags; so that, to outward appearances, the physicians are satisfied. If any poor wretch (confined and in his senses) dare complain, a score of keeper and keeperesses, that is, rogues and prostitutes, are ready to testify that it is only a 'lucid interval.' If the poor fellow becomes enraged at these falsehoods, as it is natural he should be, it immediately is set down as a proof of the truth of the keeper's assertion! A proof of this is to be had in the case of a Mr. Richards, from Birmingham. He was a young man of considerable mercantile knowledge, and had been extensively employed abroad for the house of Hope and Co., Sir Thomas Baring and Co., &c. He wrote a political pamphlet, and the Barings had him incarcerated as a lunatic, the certificate of his insanity being signed by a physician who never saw him till long after he was confined—an infamous, but a common practice! This unfortunate young man remained there for years, but he found means so make some disclosures out of doors as to in-door concerns of Hoxton mad-house, which made the owner glad to set him at liberty.

A Mr. Foster, son of the eminent and worthy Town Clerk of Liverpool, got tipsey, and wasted considerable sums of money; he was seized upon by those interested in his seclusion; his absent father was persuaded, by letters, of the truth of his son's insanity, and consented to his being locked up in Mr. Warburton's care. For a time the young man was very low, and made every effort to be released from his dungeon, but Tommy was too well paid for the bird to leave a hole in the cage by which it could escape! Young Foster saw this, and in time became reconciled to be a jail bird; he had a room assigned him, a servant to at tend upon him, wine, and other luxuries, among which, last, though not least in a young prisoner's estimation, he had the underhouse-maid, Ann, to make his bed, and share it with him! Thus was the young man's mind contaminated, and if they did not, according to their motto as before stated, 'drive him mad,' they plunged him into such a state of sensual debauchery that was, perhaps, worse than a dereliction of understanding; and his conduct served his keepers with plausible reasons to convince his friends that he was an object fit for confinement. Let any one pause for awhile upon this revolting picture, and say what he deserves who furnished materials for such a painting. Can the thing be worse?—probably, reader, you may, in your shallow judgment, think it is impossible to render it more deplorable?—you know not one tenth of the horrors these receptacles for crime inflict upon the mind and body! The young man had a wife and a child whom he tenderly loved, and he was made to believe that his wife was the cause of his confinement! when, in fact, she, at the distance of two hundred miles, believed her husband to be insane. The wife was made first miserable by a conviction of her husband's insanity—and he became a slothful, drunken, lascivious, and debauched being, rioting in a harlot's embraces, and enfeebling both his body and his soul.

When delineating the most atrocious features of this private inquisition, I am compelled to use highly respectable names: let not the blame rest upon me; I am averse to all exposures which create a pang in the feeling breast—but I sacrifice private suffering on the altar of general good. To me, it is indeed painful to record crimes that hitherto have been practised in SECRET, and are UNKNOWN, but I have a duty to do, which will, in the end, reward me for my suffering; and those who have relatives smarting under the lash of Mr. Warburton, will thank me for the discoveries I have made.

There is an old saying—'the world is not my friend, nor the world's law.' It may be justly applied to the inmates of this den of thieves, and others—for all private mad-houses are alike public evils, that should be destroyed.

WILLIAM CONGREVE ALCOCK,

Once Member of Parliament for the County of Wexford, in Ireland.

This truly unfortunate gentleman was an inmate of Whitmore House; and his place of abode, the back parlour: he was, undoubtedly out of his senses; his was

A night which knew of no returning dawn;

he would stretch his neck out of the window, and address the Speaker of the House of Commons in the language of a lunatic; and he has been beaten from that window by a weapon wielded in the hand of a brute—for such was his keeper. I qualify no crimes; I withhold no man's name from censure or praise; William Wootten, one of Warburton's most confidential scoundrels, was he that daily and nightly tormented Mr. Alcock with blows, and all the arts that a villain can conjure up to render the unhappy more miserable.

Mr. Alcock had transcient gleams of reason; there was a woman with whom he formerly cohabited; she had borne him children he wished to see her, and she him; she applied in vain for admission, and Mrs. Bruning, the Jezabel housekeeper, always said he could not be seen. I have heard Warburton say: 'By God, Mrs. Bruning, the sight of that woman would almost restore him to his senses; shut her out, damn her, shut her out!!!'

I have spoken with Mr. Alcock, and do believe a little kindness and care would have restored him to his senses; but the LASH was, like the sword of Damocles, suspended by a hair over his head, and he COUND NOT BREATHE WITHOUT A BLOW!!

Time, that wears out the traces of the deepest anguish, had its effect upon poor Alcock: he became resigned—and DIED. I will not say he was MURDERED—but he was beaten into the grave by the brawny fists of Harris, Radley, Davis, and Holl, Warburton's murdering keepers!

Often has the writer seen him KNOCKED DOWN because he did not turn in his walks when the keeper pleased!—and often has he seen his mouth stuffed with HUMAN ORDURE, in order, as Master Wootten said, to make him know good victuals when they were placed before him. The blow that caused his immediate death was occasioned by a woman; it was called an accident, and when he was confined from its effects, his keepers taunted him with merciless glee, and congratulated themselves on receiving a new suit of mourning. He died—the victim of brutality. Not alone are the persecutions of this house confined to men—the gentler sex are also subservient to worse treatment.

MISS ROLLESTON,

The daughter of Stephen Rolleston, Esq.
Chief Clerk in the Secretary of State's Office.

This amiable and interesting girl had been some time in the Asylum before I knew her; her parents were (I understood) very anxious about her recovery, and she had at intervals dawnings of reason; at these times she was admitted into the parlour, and conducted herself in such a becoming way that I am fully convinced kind treatment would have restored her to her afflicted parents *compos mentis.* Mark, reader;—a reason I give for this opinion; in her sane moments I played with her at cards, and we won; on a summer's morning, two months after, she was in the garden, and nearly frantic, the indecency of her actions was deplorable: I chanced to go out of the door as her humane friend and keeperess, Mrs. Radley, was beating her with a broom-stick on the breast; she flew to me, and said, 'Won't you save me, you know we won at cards t'other night.' I hope it is needless to say that I protected her at the moment, and conveyed her safe to her chamber, for situated as I was, neither Mr. Warburton or any of his agents were inclined to say much against my will.

Here let me pause, and calmly consider what might have been done for this wretched and amiable girl; her parents were in the highest state of affluence, and they fondly hoped, and foolishly believed Mr. Warburton could restore their lost child; they, the parents, were assiduous in their attention. I have seen and marked the anxious and enquiring eye of the father, and beheld the tear trembling in the mother's eye lids, when they have questioned Mr. Warburton 'Is she any better,' and I have felt indignant at the insidious lie that said 'she is worse than before.' Mr. Rolleston's high office may have effaced my name from his recollection, but I remember him when he was the friend of a Countess I dearly love, my noble relation; and when the person of his daughter had not been violated by the filthy dungeon villains inhabiting Mr. Warburton's mad-house.

Chance had thrown into Warburton's establishment a fellow named Kelly; he was a young man, and—but it is no matter—by the contrivance of Mrs. Bruning, the keeperess of the gaol, he slept in the same bed with Miss Rolleston, many Saturday nights. I have seen them in bed together, not once, but twenty times; and the conversation I have had with Miss Rolleston, on the subject, only convinced me of the 'damning fact', and made me sigh for the consequences of passion uncontrouled by reason. Behold, reader, a tale worthy of thy execration—I have seen the person of that child, for so I must call one bereft of reason, prostituted on the steps leading to the lodge, by more than one keeper. I have heard it mentioned to Warburton, and his answer has been, 'it is no matter; she don't know what is done to her.' I could not, at that time, take upon me to knock the villain down who used such language, revolting to human nature; but, thank Heaven, I live to record his infamy, and make the world abhor him.

I am partial to woman—who is not?—but there was something in the countenance of Miss Rolleston that pleaded for herself something that interested me towards her, and I could not tell why; something which made me pity and love the object (which for wise reasons, no doubt) was visited by the scourge of mental darkness. Mary Wilson, her keeperess, would often say, 'Go to your den, you bitch, or I'll beat your brains out.' I have given Miss Rolleston books to read, and she has said, in a tone I shall never forget till sense and memory have left me for ever, 'They have taken away the books you gave me; but give me another, and I will hide it here,' (placing her hand on her bosom). Alas, poor child of misery! thy bosom had been rifled by villains; thy treasures were stolen, and thy ways corrupted by monsters. Methinks I never saw a fairer form under the middle size—but what avails form, or face, when the gate of desolation is opened, and the ravenous wolf can prey upon the lamb without an eye to pity—an ear to hear—or a hand to defend.

Comment were almost useless, where the poor object has been prostituted in a state of death: I have no means, nor do I wish to communicate with Miss Rolleston's parents, public exposure is all I aim at, and by that I hope to accomplish a general good. A greater sink of villainy never was erected than Warburton's Mad-house. A more helpless being exists not within its walls than Miss Rolleston.

I sincerely hope that her parents may see these pages, and have her removed; no doubt Mr. Warburton will deny what I have written; he will have much to deny, for I have only just opened the door of his infamy, the interior of his den is yet to be exposed. The Augean stable, if not cleared, shall be exposed to public inspection, for I dread his enmity as little as I value his friendship; fortunately for him, Mrs. Bruning, the once famous housekeeper, the Pythoness and oracle of her master, is dead. Mr. Warburton discharged her with a small pension, and had she lived, she meant to have done what I am now doing, from different motives; she was succeeded by Miss Taylor, a girl of Warburton's, and to this concealed prostitute is confided the care of the good, the great, and the unfortunate. She is a wretch, totally void of feeling, whose aim is to make money by any means, however wicked, that lays in her power.

There is a widow of a captain of marines, whose name I have forgotten: I believe she was put into Whitmore House for getting intoxicated and abusing her neighbours, but she is no more insane than the reader. In fact, insanity is not required to gain a place in Warburton's den; he receives any one; whether fraud, malice, or self-interest prompt the relatives, it is to him a matter of no concern, and he has art to procure a physician's certificate whenever he pleases. This lady of course was strenuous in her endeavours to escape from confinement, she wrote a letter to a friend, which the keeperess found in her possession, and as a gentle admonition for her presumption, she was well flogged with a rope, and tied to her bedpost for a week, not permitting her to retire for the purposes of nature, and the stench in the room was abominable. Another attempt made by her some months after, was followed by confinement in the cellar; there she was strapped down on a tester bed, which stood betwixt two necessaries, used by all the house, being about 160 patients, and which were only emptied once a quarter; the floor was paved, and so wet, that the writer, who explored the place from curiosity, in some places got wet over his shoes; the vaulted roof was never swept, but hung with cob-webs, nor was there any light but what a small lamp afforded, which was occasionally lit at night; here a tender and delicate female was confined, and opposite to her, chained down in a similar way, was a being raving mad, whose howlings, execrations, and blasphemies continually sounded in her ears; but the hardened hearts of the keepers only laughed at this wretched woman's sufferings, and frequently left her without food for two days together, and then served her with tainted meat, and sour small beer—a slow poison, which in that house, has carried many to the grave.

The meat commonly used in this house is of the worst kind, and in summer it is often absolutely stinking: when that is the case, the poor patients get a sufficient quantity, but such as no human being would eat from choice.

In the hall there are, or was, probably forty patients; the keeper sits at the head of the table, and carves for all; no person is helped more than once, and a pint of table beer is allowed to each—in taste and effect not unlike julap and water. The meat left from the parlour table is served up in the hall, such as bones and offal, fit only for dogs.

The patients have tea in the morning, and a small slice of bread and cheese in the evening. In the front parlour are those whose friends can afford to pay most liberally; but it is a common custom to put those who are so bad as not to be likely to complain, and for whom Warburton receives the first price, into the hall, and when they are visited by their friends, they are decently apparelled, and brought into the front parlour, where their friends imagine they always reside. Wine is invariably charged to all the parlour patients, but scarcely one gets a glass except on a Sunday. In the back parlour, which is the second degree, a pint of porter is allowed to each man. This wretched beverage is made worse by the keepers, who mix it with water and stale small beer, and reserve for themselves sufficient to get drunk with every night, which is their common practice when the patients are put to bed. If the patients' friends leave them any money, the keeper takes it away the instant they are gone and those who have weekly sums are obliged to share it with their task-master.

As to work, the servants of the house do scarcely any, compelling the lunatics to wash dishes, clean knives, scour the floors, make beds, empty urinals, and do all the dirty work of the house, in which, literally speaking, more dirty work is done than meets the eye, or will bear scrutiny. I have seen Mr. Orator Hunt's brother, Mr. Gallimore, and others, beating carpets on a hot summer's day, and the keepers at the same time beating them with sticks, in order to make them work harder. The brother of Mr. Orator Hunt is more of a fool than a lunatic; he is treated like a dog, cleans the boots and shoes of the keepers, sweeps out the hall, makes up the fires, &c.—and is generally beat for his pains.

The reason given by the keepers for ill-using him is, that his brother, Mr. Orator Hunt, did not pay Warburton. I have heard them say Hunt owed £700; but for the truth of this I will not vouch, for from the first to the last, they are notorious liars: all I can say is, that this was the reason given for beating and knocking poor Hunt down, and keeping him in rags, and I think that the eloquence of his brother could not be better employed than in denouncing such receptacles as Hoxton mad-house.

There was, and may be now, for aught I know to the contrary, a Mr. Church confined; he was not mad—if he was, there was more method in his madness' than I have ever seen in any one even suspected of being *non compos mentis*; in truth, Mr. Church was a man of fortune, he had made the grand tour, and brought home all the foreign vices that degrade most of our continental travellers: he was in the habit of committing a foul of fence for which the law assigns the punishment of death, and would have been very justly banged; but Mr. Warburton's house received him as a lunatic, and saved his neck. He took advantage of a lunatic, the son of a colonel in the army, and repeatedly committed the same crime with him, in a room at the end of the house, facing the garden, occupied by a patient named Huck; no pains were taken to prevent this horrid intercourse; Mr. Church had money, which he distributed amongst the keepers, and his enormities were only talked of as things of course; yet that man sat in the front parlour, at table with men in their senses, and women too, quite capable of judging, and shuddering in the presence of such a monster. But morality never entered the head of Tom my Warburton, or any of his myrmidons. A poor wretched young girl, who was decidedly insane, and whose name I do not choose to mention, was got with child in this brothel, and the keepers used to taunt each other with being the father; the crime was laid upon one of the patients, but Mr. Warburton can, no doubt, tell who was the father if he chuses. I have heard him speak of his accident, as he termed it, with indifference, and I believe it was wholly concealed from the lady's friends.

MR. PALMER,

(Whose real name is Parnell), occupied a front room, and had a keeper entirely to attend upon him. His brother, Sir Henry Parnell,[2] Member of

---

2   Henry Brooke Parnell, 1st Baron Congleton PC (1776 – 1842), known as Sir Henry Parnell at the time, was MP for Queen's County, in Ireland, in 1801 and then from 1806 till 1832. Later, from 1836 until 1841, he would serve as Paymaster-General. It was his mentally and physically disabled brother, John Augustus, a deaf-mute, who would have otherwise inherited the family estates in 1801, but Sir Henry was allowed bypass

Parliament, paid for this servant, and also for a separate table, when in truth, he, Palmer, received his scanty meal from what was left at the parlour table, and which, when it happened to be any thing eatable for a sane person, his keeper appropriated to himself, and gave him bread and cheese.

The same keeper had a certain quantity of tea and sugar from the housekeeper every Monday morning, for his use during the week, which be sold to a person in Hoxton, and gave Mr. Palmer small beer for his breakfast. The keeper carried a small dog whip, and I have seen him beat his patient till the blood flowed from his legs, merely because he refused to go to bed before the regular time. His clothes were furnished from his brother, of the best kind, and the keeper always managed to take them away before they were worn a month, frequently demanding a new suit, alledging that he had torn the other to pieces, or burnt them.

This is commonly done by all the keepers and keeperesses throughout the mansion.

A greater robber of the poor patients did not exist than Jemmy Davis, who had charge of the Hall, and accumulated a little fortune by his atrocious peculations.

Mr. Palmer was, at length, sent over to Waterford, with a keeper, by his brother's desire, who had found out the infamous treatment he received; it would have been as well if he had punished the

him thanks to a special Act of Parliament passed in 1789. — Ed.

authors, but gentlemen hesitate before they attempt a general good when it costs them a painful family exposure.

As a proof how people are robbed and imposed upon in this brothel

MR. BEDDELL,[3]

who was put into it by Sir Francis Baring,[4] had a taste for music, he had sometimes three new piano-fortes in twelve months, it being stated that he broke them to pieces, when they were only partially injured by the keepers, and sent out and sold. The patients are always instructed to get money from their friends and visitors, to give to the keeper for his kindness; if they do not, woe be to them when they are gone.

CAPTAIN ANDERSON,

Of the Royal Navy,

Has long been an inmate of Whitmore House: he digs in the garden, wheels dung, gravel, &c., and is thrashed by the gardener to his work, as slaves

---

3   Alexander Beddell (b. 1776) was confined to Whitmore House in 1807. See George Dale Collinson, *A Treatise on the Law Concerning Idiots, Lunatics, and Other Persons Non Compotes Mentis* (London: W. Reed, 1812) 218. —Ed.

4   Sir Francis Baring, 1st Baronet (1740 – 1810), the merchant banker. —Ed.

are by negro-drivers in the West Indies. I have often heard the old man complain, but he had no friend to hear him, and is in all likelihood suffering at this time.

THE HON. AND REV. MR. BASSET,

Brother to Lord De Dunstanville[5]

Who holds a plurality of livings, has two apartments to him self; he eats and drinks luxuriously, and excepting a gouty and nervous complaint, that confines him to a rolling chair, he is as well in his health and understanding as the writer. Warburton is allowed twelve hundred pounds a year for his support. Why he is confined, I will not pretend to say; it certainly is with his own consent, and there is a mystery about him which I could probably unravel, if it were worth while to throw away time upon it. The household reports about him are what I cannot commit to writing, and should not be justified in repeating from hearsay. Lord De Dunstanville was a frequent visitor of the house, but he never saw his brother, only Warburton, with whom he had long interviews. I mention this circumstance, to show that these hous-

---

5   Francis Basset, 1st Baron de Dunstanville and Basset FRS (1757 – 1835) had, by this time, served as an MP for Penryn (a pocked borough), in Cornwall, a seat he had held until 1796. He was a partner in the Cornish Bank of Truro and chairman of the Cornish Metal Company. —Ed.

es are, in a hundred cases, mere cloaks to avoid the punishment of the law, and cheat Justice of her victim. No man would voluntarily submit to incarceration in a mad-house who possessed a handsome income, unless he had sound reasons for avoiding the eye of the world. It is needless to say Mr. Basset was well treated.

I wish Lord De Dunstanville would be candid enough to say, whether he thinks it is for the preservation of his brother's life that he is intrusted to Warburton's care.

THE REV. ROBERT CHAWNER

Was jealous of his wife, and her paramour, a man of fortune, managed with her to throw him into Whitmore House, as a lunatic. I heard a physician, to whom he had appealed as to the truth of his sanity, say: 'Pshaw! Mr. Chawner, you must be mad, or you would not be jealous of your wife.' 'If that,' said Chawner, 'is a proof of madness, then let me have the company of the Prince (now the King), for he also is jealous of his wife.'

Mr. Chawner managed, by stratagem, to escape from the house, and commenced an action for false imprisonment against Warburton, but from an error in the indictment, Warburton escaped, and Chawner did not renew the suit, though the judge advised him to do so.

The servants in this house are men of the vilest description: if they are stout able-bodied men, no question is asked where they lived, or how they lived—and the women are hired on the same terms.

One keeper, Kelly, was a deserter from the army; another had served fourteen years at Botany Bay; another was a known thief at the police offices; and seven of the keeperesses were acknowledged common strumpets, and slept with the keepers or sane patients every night, and this was sanctioned by the house keeper, old Mother Bruning.

YOUNG SIDMOUTH,

Clerk of the Pells for Ireland,

Was kept by Warburton in a separate house, and had an establishment such as it was. The chariot was only a hired one, though Lord Sidmouth paid for a new one, and actually thought his son had a handsome equipage, when he was trudging on foot, attended by a single keeper, or rolling in a hackney coach. The lady who officiated as house-keeper to this gentleman was a cast-off mistress of Warburton's, by whom he had several children. The servants, who were dressed up when Lord Sidmouth came to see his son, were only three of the lower keepers sent from Whitmore House, to appear as if they constantly attended. The chamber-maid was a strumpet, she was sent from Whitmore House for having had two bastards in the place; but it is dangerous to dismiss any one initiated in the mysteries of a mad-house; so Mr. Warburton provided for her as he had done for his mistress, at Lord Sidmouth's expence, or rather at the expence of the nation, for his son was mad when he got the appointment of Clerk of the Pells, at 3000l. a year, and will continue so till his dying day.

Lord Sidmouth is a conscientious man, yet he scruples not to rob the public, in order to pay a mad-house keeper for taking care of his son.

I believe a man named Sutherland is now keeper to the Clerk of the Pells; whether he is a relation of the Sutherland, another private mad-house proprietor, I do not know, nor is it of any importance to the facts above stated.

THE MARQUIS OF TULLIBARDINE[6]

Is treated in the same way. It does not cost £150 *per annum* to keep him, and the Duke of Athol pays Tommy more than £1000; and thus it is that the plunderers of the public are, in their turn, plundered by Warburton and his myrmidons.

To advert again to the ladies, for I profess no regularity in my account, giving what first springs to my recollection; in fact, all the cases are so bad, that it is impossible to select one less atrocious than another. The females, if there is a slight shade of difference, are worse used than the males; they are treated, even if they were really insane, with

6   John Murray, 5th Duke of Atholl (1778 – 1846), declared insane in 1798, was known by the courtesy title of Marquis of Tullibardine until his father's death in 1830. —Ed.

unnecessary harshness, an injudicious exercise of the strong arm of brutal authority, where the gentle voice of suggestion or request would have been cheer fully obeyed.

Mr. Warburton is the framer of this discipline, and if he is not fully aware of the vices of his servants, more shame for him; but he was a keeper himself, and must know their proceedings, and has not ignorance to plead in extenuation of his faults; he may try to sneak into a little credit, by cringing and smirking on the side of power, at the Pitt Club, and elsewhere; he may hug himself in his own contemptible esteem—I care not for him—-he knows that I possess the whole clue to the labyrinth of his iniquity, and he knows I have not written one word but what carries with it matter of fact.

MRS. WAKEFIELD,[7]

The authoress of many good books for little children, is frequently an inmate of Whitmore House; when she recovers, and the paroxysm goes off, she returns to society, but when she is ill they (the keepers) rob her of all she possesses. I remember—can I ever forget it?—when they stripped her in the cellar of all her apparel, which was new, and sent her up naked, all but her shift, into the parlour, pretending she had thrown them down the neces-

---

7   Priscilla Wakefield (1751 - 1832). —Ed.

sary; a new dress was ordered, and the keeperesses divided her garments amongst them.[8]

This brutal mode of robbery is frequently resorted to by those demons, and whenever a friend or relative is expected, they often dress the patient in rags, in order to have more clothes ordered.

There is no separation betwixt the women's rooms and the men's but the broken doors, they lead into the same gallery, and the patients have access to each other whenever they please. Poor Miss Rolleston one morning was found in the room of Mr. Daniels, a gentleman called to the bar, but unfortunately deranged. The keeperess, who had not sanctioned this visit, dragged her out by the hair of her head, beat her head repeatedly against the wall, and then tying her legs, flogged her as children are flogged at school, in the presence of half-a-dozen monsters in the shape of men, whose remarks at the time are too indelicate—too shocking for repetition.

This mode of punishment was often put in practice, and when the sufferer was too strong, and re-

---

8   This must have been particularly gailling given that Mrs Wakefield, a Quaker, had for years had to endure money troubles; her husband, Edward Wakefield, a prominent city merchant, gradually lost their wealth in risky investment gambles and the couple found themselves in dire straits from time to time, trying to avoid bankruptcy. They had large overheads, living in a large house at Ship Yard, off Tottenham Green. In turn, her son Daniel supplied his own share of headaches, with unhappy marriages, financial woes, and lawsuits, forcing her to take care of her grandchildren for periods of time. She wrote, in part, to support her family. —Ed.

sisted, a male was called in to assist at the revolting operation. Mr. Jemmy Davis was peculiarly active on such occasions, and seemed to take a pleasure in tormenting; he gloried in his inhumanity, with which Mother Bruning was so well acquainted, that whenever any of the patients were inclined to be obstreperous, she threatened to send Davis, and the horror of his name instantly made them quiet. The funerals from this house were always secretly conducted, and I have no doubt of the truth of the report, that the bodies were frequently sold to the surgeons.

There was also, amongst others who had no right to be in this house, a

MR. JOHN MITFORD

A relative of the Right Honourable
Lord Redesdale, and Lady Viscountess Perceval,
now Countess of Egmont

I have heard his history from his own lips, for he made no secret of it, and the correctness of his story was admitted by Mother Bruning herself, with whom he was upon the most intimate terms; whether they merited it or not, they were the talk of all that could talk reasonably in the house, but neither of them cared much about scandal, for when he chose to remain in the house, he had a young girl who visited him, as his companion; and though Mother Bruning grumbled, it was generally out of his hearing, and he certainly carried more authority than any one else presumed to do.

He, it appears, was in some situation on board a ship of war, and wishing to be free from the service, he came to town to see his relation, Viscountess Perceval, and with her Ladyship and the Princess of Wales was engaged in writing letters for the public journals, levelled at the Prince Regent, and Ministers of State: to do this more securely, and remove suspicion from the parties at Blackheath, where they were watched, their agent, Mr. Mitford, went into Warburton's, where he had an apartment, and went and came when he pleased, being always engaged in writing when within. Warburton gave him a certificate that 'he was unfit to serve in the Navy,' and he was, by this imposition, released from the service; and moreover received from the Admiralty a sum of money on account of this sham illness; I saw Mr. Warburton pay it to him—if this transaction was not swindling the Navy Office, it was close on board of it; and I don't know which to blame most of those who were connected in pursuing the deception.

It appeared the parties overleaped the bounds of prudence, and the means by which they were influencing the public mind was traced to their real source; in fact, Warburton must have been in the secret, for he knew all Mitford's concerns—knew he was visited by Lady Perceval and her agents-and he, Warburton, also went and came to and fro between Blackheath and Hoxton—be that as it may, the conspiracy was blown up, and the parties wished to shift the blame each from his own shoulders to those of his neighbour. The Princess disavowed any knowledge of the letters addressed to the public in various papers, and so did Lady Perceval, who tried to fix the responsibility upon Mitford, the scribbler, in the mad-house. The public mind was highly inflamed; and Mitford, who did not relish a prospect of the pillory, was tried in the Court of King's Bench, for letters published in *The News* Sunday paper. The Viscountess Perceval swore peremptorily that 'she only knew this Mitford as a common acquaintance, and that she knew he was not intimate with the Princess,' when, oh, dire mishap! Mr. Mitford produced a bundle of her most affectionate letters, addressed to him, which were read in court, and astonished even Lord Ellenborough,[9] when he found the lady's testimony to be 'as false as Hell;' moreover, a confidential letter from the Princess, proved to be her hand-writing, addressed to Mitford, was also read: he was acquitted; and his persecutors disgraced in every ones eyes. Mr. Warburton, at the suggestion of Lady Perceval, had said, in the daily papers, that Mitford was insane when he was drunk, which, by the bye, was pretty often. Mr. Warburton, for once, spoke truth, for was ever a drunken man yet in his sober senses.

But Warburton was too cautious; and when subpoened to swear to Mitford's insanity in court,

9   Edward Law, 1st Baron Ellenborough, PC, KC, FSA (1750 - 1818). —Ed.

he wisely kept out of the way, and left the party to make the best of what he had said, but could not swear to. Does not this very case shew that it is necessary to put down these infernal dens, even in a political point of view; here a man conspiring against the Ruler of the Kingdom, and sowing dissention amongst his subjects, was secure-no one would expect to find the companion of the Princess of Wales and Viscountess Perceval in a mad-house; and still less suspect that the letters which then teemed from the press, were the effusions of two petticoat politicians, and their convenient secretary, the sham lunatic Mitford. I believe this once celebrated champion of the Princess of Wales, and worthy relative of Lord Redesdale, is now in London; if he chooses, no one can tell more of the horrors and villanies of Whitmore House, for he was admitted into all its secret recesses, not excepting the secret recesses of the housekeeper's heart. I care no more for Mr. Mitford, than he does for me—I stand upon the solid base of truth, and am not afraid of consequences. I should be glad to know if Lord Redesdale, who is accounted a very moral and religious man, a near and dear friend to the pious Lords Sidmouth and Eldon, whether he was not privy to the deception practised by young Mitford and his party; for this I know full well, that his Lordship paid for his abode at Hoxton, and also all the expences of his trial; and I have also seen Mr. Robert Mitford, another relative of that Lord, often in close confabulation with Warburton, in the mad house.

Thus I have, I trust, made it appear that this nursery of rogues and thieves was also a focus for treason to concentrate its powers, and spread them aboad invisibly. I have been informed, that this Mitford and Warburton have ever since these events been very good friends, which rather surprises me, as Warburton was very willing to have made him appear insane, if he could have done so without committing perjury. Mr. Mitford also praised the institution in sundry letters in the public papers, and in a volume of his poetry, now in my possession, called *The Poems of a British Sailor*, he has, in a poem named 'The Maniac's Death,' lauded his friend Warburton for his humanity, and his—Mrs. Bruning, for her virtuous feeling. It is true Mr. Mitford had good reasons for this at the time—he managed, through Whitmore House, to fleece the Navy board of a pretty round sum of money, and to libel the Prince and Government in security, and for which I apprehend he was well paid.

If Mr. Mitford sees this, he will recollect his acquaintance in the Gallery, who was forcibly confined, and not a volunteer, as he was: if I have exaggerated, or told an untruth unintentionally, he knows where to find me, and is well aware that my opinion then of him, (Warburton) and his flame, Mother Bruning, was the same that is here recorded-not favourable to any one of the three and if they are dissatisfied with what I have set down, and this work goes through another edition, I will speak louder and plainer, and remind them of the girl 'Ellen,' and 'thereby hangs a tale' none of them would like to hear.

My remarks are straight forward; it is true, I cannot back them with all the influence and power which wealth gives to individuals in the present times, but they are backed by unanswerable truth.

If I am obliged to make use of names, highly respectable, and no less unfortunate, I am obliged to do so, to establish my credit for truth, without which I cannot accomplish a general good open the world's eyes to those lawless houses—and put an end to tortures and miseries that are a disgrace to this land of Christian freedom.

I attack no private character, but am obliged to produce the suffering individuals' cases to aid my attack upon the public man, and the den of horrors.

Mr. Warburton may be silent, if he pleases; no one will interpret his silence to conscious innocence; but to 'stand mute,' and not by the visitation of God, is the way many public men now support their character. This is defending your heart by holding your hands behind your back. But let me proceed: I will 'tickle your catastrophe,' my boy, before I have done with you!

Mr. Warburton 'cannot rail the seal from my bond;' no one but a person most intimate with HIM and HIS could give such a collection of NAMES, FACTS, and SECRET proceedings. I know, out of his house, he is considered a good feeling sort of man, and has many of the Royal College on his side: he may get, possibly, a dozen physicians to give him a character—but I am not accusing him of behaving ill to medical men, or being a bad neighbour, or friend, at home and in the world—it is in his public office as a mad-house keeper I accuse him of gross neglect, and unfeeling indifference to the beings under his care. He may be a very good man in parish business, and meetings at Hackney, for a man may do one thing well that cannot do another; a man may catch sparrows to admiration, when he cannot keep a secret and the medical visitors of Hoxton mad-house know nothing of its general management. Can you, Mr. Warburton, get a committee of medical men to sign their names to a denial of the specific charges herein made? No—they will not, for they conscientiously cannot. Your silence is self-condemnation—and all you have to do now, is to remain in that pristine insignificance for which the fiery ordeal I have made you go through has only rendered you a fitter subject.

But let us descend a few steps deeper into the shade of Whitmore House; let us take a view of

The cheerless tenant of the dungeon gloom;

and see if nothing more horrible than any thing I have yet advanced can be elicited from beneath the earth's surface: 'straight is the gate, and narrow is the way,' and I wish I could add, 'few there are who enter therein.' The stone steps, damp with mildew, seem to 'go down to death,' and the clanking of chains, and stifled groans, announce it as the purgatory of a living being. This dungeon, or cellar, has four apartments, under the house; one is totally unoccupied, the other full of old lumber, the third has a bed in it, where riotous patients are confined for punishment, or disobedience of the keeper's orders, and confined solely at the keeper's will; whether this power is delegated to them from their master, or they assume it of themselves, I will not take upon me to say, but I know Mr. Warburton never found fault when he knew any one was confined there and I have seen a poor wretch, for refusing to change his new shoes for the keeper's old ones, beat and lashed down on this bed, extended on his back, with his hands and feet tied to the four corner posts, and a strap drawn tight across his middle, so as to render respiration painful and difficult.

MR. RHODES,

Son of an eminent sugar-refiner near Charing Cross, has often suffered this punishment, merely for making use of unpalatable truths during his moments of unclouded reason.

MR. VIALLS,

A young man, the son of a flour merchant at Greenwich, and who had been a clerk in the East India House, had recurrences of his senses, which lasted for a day together, and during which time, the keeper was endeavouring to drive him again into a state of in sensibility, by repeating to him the actions he committed when in his raving moments, and irritating his feelings in the most inhuman way. He has repeatedly said to the writer: 'They will not let me be at peace, and I too sensibly feel I shall experience a relapse without the aid of their cruelty to hasten it.' From no cause whatever have I seen this youth, when *compos mentis*, dragged off and fastened to this bed of torture, and kept there for two days on bread and small beer. There is an aperture in the middle of the bed, and some flocks under the shoulders of the poor wretch, but no covering whatever; the window is broken, and the rain beats in upon the bedstead freely.

This is not considered as too severe a place of punishment by any keeper in the house for one that even spits upon the floor, or neglects to scrape his feet on leaving the garden. Opposite the door of this den, 'which, by the bye, was off the hinges,' are the two privies, from which arises a most intolerable smell, as there are no sewers to carry off the soil, which is suffered to accumulate till it reaches near the top, and they are full seven feet deep; I remember when they had not been emptied for six months. These places are on the left hand after you have descended the steps, and at mid-day, you must have a candle to find them out—which you cannot do by the smell, as that pervades every part of this dungeon, and every gasp of breath draws in pestilence and pollution. Betwixt those receptacles is a small room, in which a wretched old man was constantly confined. I have been assured that he was seven years there without seeing the light of the sun; a glimmering of day indeed came in through a broken casement, just sufficient to enable you to distinguish the gloomy horrors of the place, and render imprisonment more dreadful. There was much secrecy observed about this isolated being, I was six months acquainted with the house before I knew the extent of his punishment; he was generally kept extended on the bed, and had his hands loosened when he took his meals. Mr. Davis, after dinner in the hall, collected the scraps into a dish or bowl, and taking a large leather belt in his hand, proceeded to his victim, exclaiming 'I always has to beat the wittals into the obstinate———' I have heard his shrieks, in spite of the doors being closed, when they went to administer the dose to this child of affliction. I never saw him but once, he had a few rags to cover his body, such as an old coat and trowsers; his beard was of a patriarchal length, matted, and grey; his eyes filled with glutinized rheum, and his form a skeleton; his arms and hands, looking like eagles legs and talons, dark bony, and shrivelled. Fortunately for him, a discovery was made, if I recollect right, of an American, who had been confined and tortured in Bethnal Green mad-house, and the indignation of the public was roused against such inquisitions. This alarmed Mr. Warburton and his satellites; the poor wretch was released from his bed, a worse than 'Damien's bed of steel,' because its torture was unending; he was shaved, washed, decently apparelled, and removed in the dead of the night to another of Warburton's mad-houses, (for he has shares in many) and I learnt from a keeper, who was too humane to hold his place long, that he was permitted to walk in a large gallery, was perfectly harmless, and comfortable. This indulgence might, with attention, perfectly cure him; no doubt, he was always a lunatic, but it is no reason, admitting that he was a lunatic of the most dangerous description, that he should be buried in filth, shut out from the light of heaven, and treated worse than a beast of prey—who, at least, can roam at large in its den, and rise up and lay down at its pleasure.

Shortly after this man's removal, the whole mansion was cleaned and fumigated—the patients better clad and fed—the cellar windows mended—and the dungeons made decent—the beds or bedsteads being repaired—and the night soil removed. This was preparatory to a very narrow inspection which the visiting physician's made. The patients are then asked if they have any complaints to make of the victuals or the treatment? If a man is mad it is obviously a folly to question him thus; if he be in his senses, and the physicians believe his replies, whether for, or against the establishment, they ought to order his discharge, as an unfit subject for controul; but I never knew this to be done. A Mr.

Richards, whom I before mentioned, as being confined by the house of Baring and Co. upon this occasion appealed to the physicians, but the housekeeper testifying 'that he was not always so quiet;' he remained without redress, and all his rational reasoning was only considered as the cunning of a mad man.

At the time Mr. Mitford was alledged to be so diseased in his mind that he was 'unfit to serve His Majesty as an officer at sea,' for such was the tenor of the certificate sent by Mr. Warburton to the Lords of the Admiralty, he was writing the incendiary letters, signed 'Matthew Bramble,' which appeared in *The Star* newspaper, and jointly with his relative and friend, Viscountess Perceval, those signed 'Justicia,' for which she was exposed in court, and compelled to acknowledge; and I should be glad to know if any one, who had read those able productions in a wrong cause, can see any proofs of a diseased mind in the forcible and eloquent language Mr. Mitford there uses with the dexterity of an able advocate. Moreover, it was signified to Mr. Warburton that a naval physician would see Mr. Mitford, and when he came, he was taken up stairs to the room of an insane patient, since dead, who was pointed out to him by Mr. Warburton as Mr. Mitford—the latter standing by as a friend to witness this personation of himself. The consequence was, the deceived physician granted instantly a certificate of Mitford's insanity, which was backed by Mr. Warburton, who forwarded it to the Admiralty, and Mitford, in a few days, received his discharge, and a liberal sum of money in compassion for his sufferings.

The physician thus imposed upon, I am pretty confident was Dr. John Weir. That day, Mr. Mitford dined with Mr. Warburton, and in the evening, accompanied by a young lady, who visited him often, he went to the theatre, and did not return again for several days, when he came accompanied by the Viscountess Perceval, and several friends, no doubt to congratulate with Warburton on the success of their scheme, and laugh at the wise acres of the Admiralty. It is not my business to account for this proceeding being acquiesced in by Mr. Mitford; but it appears by a pamphlet, published by Mr. Phipps, the editor of the 'News,' that he was so attached to the Viscountess Perceval, she could make him consent to any thing she pleased. I hope it was so for he appeared to me a very gentlemanly young man, and I have cheered the solitude of my incarceration in Whitmore House many an hour in his agreeable company, and I know that he greatly exerted himself to obtain the discharge of young Mr. Foster, son of the Town-Clerk of Liverpool, and Mr. Chawner, the clergyman, who were both unjustly confined.

Here, reader, I have stated a strong case, and if Mr, Warburton can conscientiously deny—but I beg pardon, I never supposed him to have any conscientious feelings, and am going to give him credit for that to which he is a total stranger. In this case, the Government of the country were completely tricked, and whatever pay or pension Mr. Mitford now enjoys has been obtained under false pretences. I say so boldly, and am not afraid of either Mr. Warburton or Mr. Mitford proving that I say wrong. I defy them to do it. There is no deception but what may be practised under cover of these houses.

Mr. Warburton also sends keepers to all parts of the kingdom, and when he has not room in his house, he secures his patients in private lodgings. He had several lodged at and near Kingsland Crescent, amongst them the Marquis of Tullibardine. His keeperess was a strumpet, and I have had the honour of sitting at table, and spending some evenings with her and her bastards in Warburton's parlour. She made a fine harvest of her patient, who, by-the-bye, was no more insane than the Duke of Athol himself. At these times, when the keeperess came to visit Mrs. Bruning, and spend a merry day, (for the lady was particularly partial to Holland's gin, and generally poured down so many libations to the gods, that before it was time to depart, she was unable to go unsupported), at these times, her noble patient, the Marquis, was left at the porter's lodge, inside the gate, where, in the society of the porter, and sundry keepers, he smoked his pipe, and enjoyed his gin and porter as well as he could.

The lady keeperesses also come in for their share of plunder, and they managed amongst them

to strip him of all his spare cash. The noise issuing
from this lodge, by singing obscene songs, could
be distinctly heard in the housekeeper's parlour,
and Mr. Warburton himself often passed it unnoticed at these times. Can the reader reflect without
indignation at such vile proceedings? Here was
a situation for the heir to 'the King of Mona!' the
first-born son to Athol's mighty duke, to whom Mr.
Pitt presented fifty thousand pounds of the public
money, cooped in the corner of a porter's lodge,
associating with rogues and strumpets, swallow-
ing gin and beer, while his keeperess was performing the same vile deeds within, on a somewhat
higher scale. Confinement, and the society of such
wretches, had deadened the feelings, and stupified
the senses of this Marquis, who was sure daily to
get worse under the care of his keepers.

The Duke of Athol, I apprehend, has a partiality
for mad-houses; he had a Lady Murray once confined for some foolish reason, and probably would
confine his other son,[10] if he could catch him, who
is rambling on the continent, on the paltry pittance
of 600l. *per annum*: if his grace possesses no feeling for his son, and has so little hereditary Scotch
pride belonging to him, as not to feel hurt at this,
and apply the remedy that is in his power, perhaps
his hereditary meanness and penurious disposition will be exerted to save a penny, when I assure
him that his son would be better treated and more

10   Lieutenant-General James Murray, 1st Baron Glenlyon KCH
      FRS (1782 – 1837), styled Lord James Murray until 1821. —Ed.

respectably attended by an honest man and woman, for one hundred pounds a year, than he is in his present state for one thousand.

I have already stated the case of a Miss Rolleston somewhat at large, and could give that of many other females, equally desirable of being made known; but I hope enough has been said to awaken suspicion in the minds of those who have relatives in this den of horrors, that they might be better treated if they believed less of the keepers' assertions than formerly, and that the only cure for insanity at Whitmore House is—death.

I am induced to give one more case of a female, and shall particularise no other. This lady had been a dweller in darkness for some years, and was apparently about twenty-five or twenty-six years old; she was a harmless lunatic, dressing herself up with flowers, carrying a basket of them, and chanting simple songs, at intervals, as she repeatedly paced the galleries or the garden; they called her 'Crazy Jane,' and that was the only name I ever knew her by; she was very pretty, but with all that wildness of appearance about her, which Shakespeare has given to Cassandra, the inspired denouncer of the fate of Troy. One morning she was walking the gallery at an early hour, when a keeperess asked her what right she had to be out of her room without permission, and proceeded to snatch from her the basket of flowers—tear her cap from her head—and strike her in the face with clenched fists till the blood came; the poor creature fell down on her knees and begged for mercy, when she kicked her backwards by a blow in the stomach, where she lay insensible. A person, whose name I do not chuse to mention, knocked down this humane keeperess, and then kicked her down the first flight of stairs; he then reed the pitiable object of her brutality into the ladies' apartment, and by the aid of a woman less ferocious, restored her to life. The housekeeper was made acquainted with this atrocious transaction, and pertly remarked that the keeperess knew her duty, and Crazy Jane was a devil if she was not kept under: not satisfied with this, the same person mentioned it to Mr. Warburton, who said he would allow none of the female patients to be beat out of their room—a tacit admission that the torture in secret might be applied as severely, and as often as the heartless beings called keeperesses chose to inflict it. This poor maniac this Crazy Jane, had sufficient beauty to attract the eyes of the keepers, and was made the victim of their lust; and I have often seen her hurried by them down into the cellar, before I knew the horrid purposes for which it was done. That she had some feeling I know—but whether bodily or mental sufferings brought it forth I am ignorant, though in either case it is dreadful to think of; for I have seen her hurry tottering up the cellar steps, from that cavern of pollution, her eyes streaming with tears, which she tried to hide as she ran into the garden. And at such times I have seen her beaten, the keeperess declaring she could not keepher from the men—a burning lie to my certain know ledge; depraved in themselves, they knew not what virtue meant, and the sacred stream of pity never flowed in their corrupt veins. Mr. Chawner, the clergyman, once emphatically denounced those women to the housekeeper as the sweepings of Hell, if so, it is a pity that place should ever be swept; at all events, they are the scum of the earth, and were the kennels of St. Giles's to be raked for infamy, none would be found to equal them; yet they dressed well, and could assume a look of cheerful humility, and shew tenderness to their patients when occasion called for them thus to do penance to the real sentiments of their base hearts. I have seen them receive presents from the afflicted friends for their kindness, when those, from whom they received this reward, were worse used by them than any others.

One afternoon, Miss Rolleston ran up stairs before the house keeper in a rude romping way, as might be expected from her situation. The old lady, to teach her respect, as she said, ordered her to be straight waistcoated; it was hardly done before her parents came, when the old sycophant herself brought her down stairs into the parlour neatly dressed, and received from her mother, as a reward of her humanity, a silk dress, and when they were gone, she laughed at their folly, and ordered the punishment of the waistcoat again to be inflicted on the poor girl, unconscious of having given any offence.

There was a lady confined by her husband, labouring under melancholy madness, or rather a powerful nervous complaint; he called every Sunday to see her, and she always entreated him with tears, to have her removed, but gave no reason why she wished it, and the keeperess took care they should never be alone together, from fear that she might tell 'the secrets of her prison house.'

One day he suddenly appeared, and reluctantly they were forced to bring her down; she had two black eyes, her cheeks were swollen, and her arms black and blue with pinches; her husband sent for a coach, and instantly removed her. The establishment were all alarmed, and how it was settled I never heard: but Mr. Jemmy Davis told me afterwards, with exultation in his countenance, that she was dead at another house, and he was d——d glad of it, for she had tried to give their's a bad name; but the mind sickens at the repetition of such horrors, and I sometimes ask myself, if I live and breathe—am of the same flesh—and am formed by the same hand which gave life to these monsters. Successful guilt makes her votaries think themselves innocent, and I doubt not but Jack Ketch deems his occupation as honourable as it is necessary; and truly, when compared to the myrmidons in Whitmore House, Jack Ketch suffers an injustice, for he has not the power of life and death in his hands, but is only the passive instrument in the hands of justice. These wretches have the power of life and death in their hands—to give or take in secret, by slow or quick means, as they please, and it is dreadful to reflect upon it—trust the hare in a kennel of hounds—place the lamb under the paw of the lion—or the young fawn in the quivering lips of the blood-reeking tyger; there are more hopes of mercy for these, than for those bereft of reason, under the human butchers in a private mad-house.

Various are the modes of torture applied, according to the whim or caprice of a keeper. One of the patients was termed a half witted fellow, like the brother of Orator Hunt: he was a harmless fool, and if all such were confined, ten thousand plough tails in the country at this time would want followers. This youth was fond of smoking, and had a certain quantity of tobacco sent him by his friends; the keeper seized it as his prey, and supplied him from the garden with Stramonium, which used in this way, is sure to produce mental derangement. I pointed out to the keeper the dangerous consequences of persisting in this, the reply was worthy of the demon that uttered it—'I give it him on purpose to make him madder, and then I'll lock him up for good and be rid of him'—can any thing be more horrible than this deliberate mental murder?

That the patients in Mr. Warburton's other houses were worse used (if possible) than in this, I have reason to believe, as the keepers threatened to send theirs to the White House, where they would find a difference, and moreover, all the refuse that remained when the vegetables were selected for Whitmore House such as cabbage leaves, and damaged potatoes, with meat that had been kept too long, were packed in a cart, and sent to other houses.

I once asked Mrs. Bruning if it was possible such stuff was going to human beings for consumption. 'Oh,' said she, 'Mr. Warburton has plenty of parish patients, and it is good enough for them, for they don't bring in more than eight shillings a week in the lump.' The sour small beer was also sent for the same purpose, and I trust, if there are parishes who farm their insane poor out to private mad-house keepers, they will attend to this hint, and see that they are not fed upon what would disgust a brute, or rather slowly poisoned by avaricious and inhuman monsters.

Some people derive both profit and fame from the dwellers in mad-houses. I will mention one curious circumstance, merely to show, beyond contravention, that I am perfectly acquainted with every wheel that moves this enormous machine and the streams which feed it from outside.

MR. JOHNSON,

A Scotchman of much learning, the author of the *History of Shetland*, and other very valuable works, from a long course of severe study has become hypochondriacal, and imagines that he would be insane if not under Warburton's care.

He pays one hundred a-year for his board and a room to study and sleep in. He labours incessantly for the booksellers, and seldom goes abroad, except from necessity as far as Paternoster Row, to settle accounts and get books. He compiled, with uncommon care and labour, in twelve months, *The Statistical History of Ireland*,[11] so often quoted in parliament and our courts of justice, and which has the name of Mr. Wakefield,[12] the Chancery lawyer, attached to it as the author, who only furnished notes and received copy.

I do not mention this to deprive Mr. Wakefield of his borrowed plumes, but to convince Mr. Warburton that I possess the clue of Ariadne to wind through every maze of his labyrinth, and could, if I pleased, and saw any good to be accomplished thereby, give a list of names, and the sums paid by the friends of a hundred patients under his care. One thing let me ask him: why is there always an apothecary's bill charged on account of a patient who never takes medicine?—is it because Mr. Dunston, the house-surgeon and apothecary, is his son-in-law, and calls once a-week to ask the housekeeper how she does? Pray, Mr. Warburton, did not you charge Lord Redesdale ninety pounds for medicine given to Mr. Mitford, when the only medicine he took was a little bark and port wine, occasionally,

---

11 The work is in fact *An Account of Ireland, Statistical and Political* (London: Longman, Hurst, Rees, Orme, and Brown, 1812). —Ed.

12 Edward Wakefield (1774–1854). —Ed.

to qualify the hot punch enjoyed by him and Mrs. Bruning over their evening card table.

Was not the same done by young Foster and Richards and Daniels. Shame on such extortions. Apropos of

MR. DANIELS;

He is, too, a harmless lunatic, whose only amusement was strumming on an old piano-forte in the front parlour. He had a sister who anxiously and attentively visited him. When she was absent, Daniels was either locked up in his room in the gallery, in the middle of winter, without a fire, or turned into the garden with scarce any covering to his body, and repeatedly horsewhipped, because he was obstinate, and spoke contemptuously of the keepers. The morning that his sister was expected, he was dressed, drank tea in the parlour, had a trifling thing given him to keep him in temper, and she generally found him at the piano, apparently tranquil. Deception, all is deception and refined cruelty, from the master down to the cook in the kitchen, who, when a patient intruded upon her premises, flung a saucepan, filled with boiling water in his face, that completely deprived it of the skin, and nearly obliterated the sight of one of his eyes. Yet, reader, was the being who thus suffered, a harmless, inoffensive, gentlemanly man, the brother to one Hawkes, a very rich coal-merchant in the city. He had been a Lieutenant Fire Worker in the East Indies, and his name has been honourably mentioned in the Gazettes as a gallant and brave officer. He was struck with a '*a coup de soleil*,' more commonly known as 'a stroke of the sun.' Warburton had one hundred and fifty pounds *per annum* for his support. Fifty pounds would have allowed his keeper a fair profit, and kept him comfortable, when all that he got for the larger sum was an extra beating from the merciless fangs of Jemmy Davis, when he amused himself by marching up and down the room in military style.

Poor Captain Johnson, whom I have before mentioned as having been nineteen years confined, was informed by Warburton, that the last of his relations was dead, and had left scarce sufficient to support him, so that he must be removed to a cheaper place. A cheaper place, reader, than the hall of Whitmore House, where no one costs, upon an average, one shilling *per diem*. Habit had reconciled this respectable old man to his situation, and he naturally wished to die for ever where he had suffered a living death of nineteen weary years: he pleaded in vain—it was the robin pleading for release under the claws of the vulture. He offered even to work in the garden, or do any thing. No; Warburton was inflexible—his laws more cruel than those of the Medes and Persians; or, to use a merited comparison, like those of Draco, the Athenian lawgiver, which were said to he written in blood, were not to be altered, and the miserable heart-broken being was taken to the White House, Bethnal Green, where a broken heart has perhaps, e'er this, terminated his journey through a long blank wilderness of woe.

The reader may think common humanity should have induced the keeper to comply with an old prisoner's desire, to die where he had lingered and suffered; but what will he think of outraged humanity, when I tell him he had a right to comply with his desire—that the person who died had left an annual sum, amply sufficient to keep poor Johnson in comfort all his future days, and that he was removed amongst parish paupers, whilst the money went to swell the hoard of him whose god was Mammon—whose will was law—and that law injustice.

MR. WILKINSON,

Who wrote *The History of the Caucasian Mountains*,[13] and had travelled over Europe and Asia, was a poor weak mortal, not able to stand on his legs for any time; he had books sent by his relatives to amuse him; when any book was well bound, or valuable, the keepers, when he was in the garden, drove him from the seat where he was, and com-

---

13   There is a work titled *A General, Historical, and Topographical Description of Mount Caucasus*, 2 vols. (London: C. Taylor, 1807), whose title page shows Charles Wilkinson as the translator. The authors are Jacob Reineggs and Freiherr Friedrich August Marschall von Bieberstein. —Ed.

pelled him to walk about: to conciliate them he would give up his book, which was immediately sold to a Jew, and gin purchased with the money. Another

MR. WILKINSON

Rider to a tea warehouse, for some imprudence committed ready receptacle—this sepulchre, which received in its remorseless jaws every one without distinction, and of which it might be said—

> Alas! from whence there's no retreating,
> Alas! from whence there's no return.

Mr. Wilkinson soon recovered from the effects of his intemperance, and repeatedly wrote to his father in the country, entreating an order for his release, but always received evasive replies; he consulted me, and I saw from the tenor of these letters, that those to his father had either been altered, or never sent by Warburton, and that his family were ignorant of his situation. I wrote to his father a true statement of his case, and in a few days he came to London and took his son away, refusing to pay a single shilling for his unjust detention. Mr. Wilkinson opened business on his own account, in Basinghall-street, and is now prosperous and happy, after so narrow an escape from confinement for life.

MRS. SCARRON,

A most respectable lady, was a parlour boarder, and had been so for years: she was accomplished, sensible, and modest: her husband confined her only because he wanted to get rid of her: she was reconciled to her situation, and looked to the grave as the only prospect of future happiness.

MRS. WILSON,

And several other ladies, were in possession of reason, but locked up with maniacs of the worst description; shut out from all hope, and unnoticed and unknown were bending broken hearted over an early tomb.

I could mention many more, such as Mr. Blagrove, Mr. Daniels, Mr. Bogg, Mr. Carter, &c. all quiet beings, yet who were disciplined with the lash, and cruelly treated, never knowing an interval of ease, except when a relation came to see them,

MR. JOHNSON

Once escaped, but was brought back, and so rigorously treated, that he declared he never would risk such an attempt again. His confinement had lasted nineteen years, and will only terminate with his existence. But it is useless for me to enumerate more instances than I have done, to show that a Private Madhouse is worse than an Inquisition, and should not be permitted in a free country; in six cases out of ten the individuals are confined from malice, or interested motives on the part of their connexions; many are confined to escape the punishment due to their crimes; and the truly insane are punished as though the affliction sent by heaven, was a crime against the world's law, and the world's creator.

I have some reason to fear that this house, bad as it appears in these pages, is one of the best regulated near the metropolis. Imagine to yourself, reader, something worse, if you can, and then nature will shudder at the reflection, that such a thing exists as a hell upon earth, for the protection of the guilty and the scourge of the innocent. How comes it that such houses are permitted by the authorities to exist, if his majesty's subjects are not protected in them—for the act that deprives them of reason, does not deprive them of their civil rights—they are the more entitled to protection from being the less able to protect themselves. Is it not as bad to connive at the existence of brothels, as unblushingly to license Private Mad-houses, for they are both receptacles of vice, crime, and erring reason. If they are suffered to continue, it is the duty of the Crown to look more narrowly into those legalized establishments, and cause mercy to ameliorate the prisoners' sorrows, and throw the light of hope upon the dark gloom of the secret dungeon.

The advocates for the extinction of foreign slavery, will do well to look at home—to the slavery of the Whites, in Private Mad-houses; there they are worse treated than negroes—the maniacs are there abused as an inferior cast of beings; as a degraded and malignant race, and they are made so by cruel treatment. Surely amongst the men of rank, honour, and wealth I have mentioned, and who have relatives suffering the torments of the damned, some one will be found to step forth, and call the attention of the legislature to the reformation of these crying evils—but if none can be found manly enough to attempt a public good, they have it in their power to privately benefit the hapless beings confined, and dear to them by the ties of blood, country, or friendship. For mine own part, I rejoice at the resolution I took to get through this painful work—this appeal in behalf of those who cannot appeal for themselves; it has long occupied my attention, and I have done it but feebly—but the simple truth is superior to eloquence in rousing the feeling hearts of sensible men, to pity those whose mental darkness is deplorable, and who are capable of enjoying no comforts beyond those of present bodily ease, and sufficient nourishment to prevent starvation.

Another important feature of these Establishments is, that they protect men from the laws who are guilty of detestable offences, for which the punishment of death is a poor atonement. They encourage the bold and adventurous to rob their neighbours and relatives, whom, upon the signature of two men, they may immure for life: and they afford a protecting shelter for those perturbed spirits who sow sedition over the land, and from their secret cavern promote anarchy and confusion by which they hope to obtain the pecuniary reward for insidious villany.

If I have given any one feeling bosom pain, in the course of this little narrative, I am sorry for it, having studied to mention families or names no more than was absolutely necessary to give effect to this exposure of the Horrors of a Private Mad-house, and rouse an abler advocate to reform them. If I succeed, by this attempt, in removing a chain from the leg of one sufferer—of suspending the lash, wielded in vengeance over the innocent head of one poor victim—of preventing the violation and degrading treatment of one unfortunate female, I shall think myself happy, and under the self-approbation of my conscience, defy the threats of a wealthy petty tyrant and merciless oppressor.

FINIS

PART SECOND

OF THE

CRIMES AND HORRORS

IN THE INTERIOR OF

WARBURTON'S PRIVATE MAD-HOUSE

AT

HOXTON AND BETHNAL GREEN;

AND OF THESE ESTABLISHMENTS IN GENERAL,

WITH REASONS FOR

Their Total Abolition

ALSO AN ACCOUNT OF THE MANNER OF TREATING HIS LATE MAJESTY,
BY WARBURTON'S KEEPERS; AND THE DISMISSAL OF DAVIS

FOR KICKING AND STRIKING THE KING!

DEDICATED TO

THE LORD CHANCELLOR,

AND

THE HONOURABLE HENRY GREY BENNETT, MP

BY

JOHN MITFORD, ESQ.

'Crimes follow crimes, and meet the astonished eye,
As to the traveller Aps on Apls arise.'

London
Spradabach Publishing
2023

To

The Lord Chancellor Eldon,
Hereditary Keeper of the King's Conscience;
and Keeper of Lunatics in General;

AND

The Honourable Grey Bennett, M.P.

I DEDICATE THIS BOOK

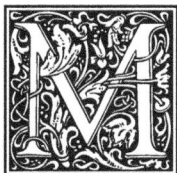

y Lord,—When I inscribe this Work with your name, it is from no feelings of respect towards you in your high station, or your private character as an individual; in truth, there is no book so worthless but I think would suffer in general estimation by having the name of John Scott on its title page; but the subjects here descanted upon, it is a part of your duty to investigate; to correct the abuses of these horrible inquisitions, and rescue the martyrs therein from tortures worse than the flames of Smithfield, or Damien's bed of burning steel.

If you are really ignorant of the facts contained in this book, it is no discredit to you; for previous to

Part First being published, the public were in total ignorance of the magnitude to which tyranny had arrived almost within sight of the powers of legislation; but that there are Private Mad-houses you must have known, from the son of your sanctified friend, Sidmouth, being a tenant of one, and you were one of the Privy Council who bestowed upon that insane boy Three Thousand a Year of the Public Money, as a Clerk of the Pells in Ireland!!! You have now, my Lord, two books before you, filled with an account of the Crimes and Horrors in these houses, to which you ought to bend an enquiring eye; and over the individuals confined, hold a protecting arm. The duties of your high office are, no doubt, heavy, and so is the purse you annually fill for performing them. You are a conscientious man, filled with tremblings and doubts on all occasions; there is no doubt, my Lord, but it would prove a balm to your conscience, if you would not shut your ear to the prisoners' cries; and where

Suffering Virtue bleeds and pines,

Let your mercy extend. Your power is very great, and it cannot be exercised to a better and nobler purpose than relieving the captive confined without just cause; turning the rod of the oppressor upon himself, and preventing any private Bastilles being kept, into which a freeborn British subject can be plunged, upon the Lettre de Cachet of one interested physician.

My Lord, this is your duty. You are growing old in doubt and indecision; take up this matter from your heart, and the recollection will relieve the horrors of a doubting death-bed, and clear your views to another world by the sweet reflection of having done your duty in this, to the best of your judgment, to the poor and afflicted.

My Lord if you take our advice, it will redound to your honour. We never had a good opinion of your tenderness of heart; we shall be glad to record, that in your old age, you have given us just cause to change it for a better.

MR. BENNETT

We have associated your name with that of John Scott, because we wished not to divide our Dedication; and your name is so highly respected, it will not for once suffer by being in his company. We earnestly and respectfully recommend to your reflection this Work; it is a cause worthy the exercise of your talents in behalf of suffering humanity. You have already done much—a glorious scene now lies before you to break the fetters laid by Villainy upon Innocence; set the prisoner free; emancipate Englishmen from private lawless dungeons; and, above all, render as happy as possible those hapless beings upon whom hope never dawns, and the light of reason never smiles.

The statements in this Work, Sir, are all true, and not exaggerated; and those by whom they are given, are ready in any place to attest their validity.

We have hopes, Sir, that this Dedication to you will be given to a good purpose, and expect to see the abuses in Private Madhouses remedied in a place where the power to remedy exists, and you have the power to set it in motion.

I am, with respect,

My Lord ELDON's Free-Admonitor,

AND

Mr. GREY BENNETT's obedient Servant,

THE PUBLISHER
Byron's Head,
Castle Street, Leicester Square.

Warburton's
Private Mad-Houses,

Whitmore House, Hoxton, White House, Bethnal Green, &c. &c.

Fie on't! 'tis a rank unweeded garden;
Things rank and gross in nature possess it.
Shakespeare

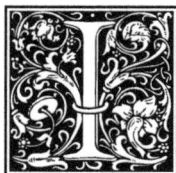

I t was the remark of an ancient philos-
opher, that he considered himself still
ignorant when any thing remained for
him to learn; and Julius Cæsar said,
he looked upon it that he had gained
nothing, whilst aught remained to conquer. So, in
a humbler way, but not less sincere, we shall never
be satisfied that our end is accomplished, whilst one
notorious case of injustice remains to be exposed;
nor till we have driven these petty tyrants from their
strong holds, and seen the day when—

Prone to earth oppression shall be hurl'd,
Her name, her nature wither'd from the world.

The sensation created by the First Part of our Work has not subsided; nor will it subside, whilst in the breasts of men one spark of love, humanity, or pity remains. We have had threats, hopes, and promises held out to us in vain; we are not to be bullied, preached, or flattered out of a thing which we have taken up from motives of conscientious feeling; and nothing can disturb our operations; we will keep the even tenor of our way, and neither deviate to the right hand or to the left, unless called aside by truth and justice. If we wanted any testimony more gratifying than universal approbation, we have had it, in the numerous private testimonials borne to our correctness, by individuals who have writhed under the lash, or fallen beneath the Herculean clubs of Warburton's cruel Alguazils in his British Inquisitions. Many of them are now moving in rank and respectability, and we have authority to give their cases in this work, which will cause

> Each particular hair to stand on end,
> Like quills upon the fretful porcupine.

We have recorded, and are proceeding to record scenes at which many a father's blood will boil, and many a tender mother's eyes be dimmed with

> Tears, such as angels weep,

Over the child they loved; and on which they

would not permit the winds of heaven to breathe too roughly.

Proceed, reader, we will surpass thy expectation. The road is flinty, and tracked with blood—but pursue it in humanity's cause with us, to rescue suffering virtue from the dungeon, and bring the jailors to the judgment of public opinion.

Let us introduce our readers into the cemetery of Whitmore House through the unhappy medium of a woman; over whose head the blast of calamity had passed with ruthless vengeance; who had seen bright and brilliant days—had lived in splendour as the wife of a man who had fought for his country, and closed a life ennobled by honourable deeds, on the field of glory—he breathed his last sigh at the battle of Alexandria, and left his wife a legacy to his country, and a prey to villains. The name of Colonel Ellis can never be forgotten on the annals of fame neither shall the name of his unfortunate wife be soon forgotten, but her memory be deplored and avenged, if the pen of simple truth can awaken the tear of sympathy, or rouse a British heart at her mournful tale. Let Mr. Warburton read and wonder, and probably fear, when I mention the name of POLL; for this, in Whitmore House, was the *nom de guerre* of

MRS. HESTER ELLIS

Even he will not be able to find out how I came by her real name and history. Let him read if he dare, and he will know what all the world shall know. This woman was, in her husband's life-time, a resident in Ely Place, Holborn; and she was a daughter of Admiral Winter. She had been introduced at the British court, and moved in the first circles, and was once looked up to with enquiring eyes as

The glass of fashion and the mould of form.

Her husband fell, and her fortunes with him. The pension of a colonel's widow, and £200 per annum were all she inherited; for his was but life property, and the life of a soldier is an honourable though a frail security. For reasons which I neither know or care, she quarrelled with her relatives; her brother and sister-in-law threw her into Warburton's, and seized upon her property. She told me, and I have no cause to doubt her truth, that government paid an additional sum towards her confinement on account of her being the widow of a gallant officer; whilst she had a private fortune, to enable her relations to receive which, every half year Warburton presented her papers, she was from fear, obliged to sign. I saw Mrs. Bruning once present her three papers to sign, and she said, 'this is cruel indeed; I will not sign.' Mrs. Bruning, with a terrible frown, and significant nod, handed the papers to a keeperess, and in a few minutes they came down to the parlour, signed, no doubt, as they pleased Mrs. Bruning, and she rewarded the keeperess with a glass of brandy.

Mrs. Ellis had a son abroad; and I occasionally saw her in the gallery, and had promised to assist her efforts to escape, by delivering a letter to some one in Bedford Row, but her sudden illness prevented me. She was a woman apparently about fifty years of age, but time had

> ——thinn'd her flowing hair,
> And bent her with his iron hand.

She bore no trace of her early beauty, except the fading lustre of her intelligent blue eyes; which, to my mind, conveyed the painful intelligence that she was dying of a broken heart. I cannot say I ever saw her used ill—except oaths and threats are called ills in a Private Madhouse—but she was evidently unjustly confined; and in her senses daily fed, and nightly locked up with raving lunatics, in a place where

> By the bonds of Nature feebly held,
> Minds combat minds, repelling and repell'd,
> Till over-wrought the general system feels,
> And motion stops, or frenzy fires the wheels.

On the morning that terminated all her earthly sufferings, and rescued another victim from the tormentors' fangs, her son arrived; he was dressed in the uniform of some dragoon regiment; and seemed deeply distressed. He was talked over by Warburton, on the Green; and was certainly not aware of the treatment his mother had experienced. Reader! what must have been this son's feelings, when returning from the field of danger with a little fortune gained in the cannon's mouth, in hopes to kiss her lips that had often breathed a prayer for him as he slept unconscious in the cradle—to find those lips pale—those eyes that always beamed upon him with affection—dim; and that forehead beneath whose covering of dark ringlets his innocent hands had often played—covered with the damp dews of a premature death, brought on by torture; to find, surrounded by filthy dungeon villains, robed in rags, the mother of his heart in the guilty walls of a private madhouse; lying stretched on the final bed of human misery—oh! what must have been his feelings?—my pen fails—nay, the pen of the eloquent apostle Paul had failed to do justice to the scene; but the breathless anxiety of a despairing child has registered the deed in heaven, where the doers will one day receive sentence. Surely there is a life beyond the grave; and a presiding spirit that leads us on earth; or why do I write? I, the child of ignorance and adversity; incapable of making a just grammatical pause, or balancing a single sentence; something leads me on, and fancy tells me I am, perhaps, laying the cornerstone of a temple, which hereafter may rise sacred to humanity and British honour, over the ruins of Private Mad-houses, which are a terror to human nature, and a disgrace to England!

Let me, for a moment, run back on the wheels of retrospection to long past ages; to the history of nations, whose proudest monuments the hand of Time has crumbled into dust; whose mountains have been removed from their base, and whose streams have recoiled to the source from whence they sprung-they had their laws for the reward of virtue, and the punishment of vice—the Parthian placed the victim upon harrows; the Persian exposed him to the burning sun; beneath whose scorching rays his bones were whitening, whilst his heart was warm within. The Druid of Britain made his human sacrifice in a wicker cage over a slow fire. The Vestal of Rome, no longer a virgin, was plunged into a cavern, with a pale lamp, and a pitcher of water. The lamp destined to burn when her lamp of life was extinguished; the pitcher of water ready to afford her a cooling draught when the parched tongue was riveted between the death-clenched teeth, and she felt the pangs of thirst no more. All these punishments sound horrible, but they were just-the victims were guilty of crimes, and were amenable to the punishment decreed by the laws of their country, and which they had no right to break, whether they were founded in ignorance or superstition. But it remained to an age when every heart was enlightened by the truths of the gospel, to condemn a man unheard, and punish him without crime. It was left to Great Britain, the chartered land of freedom—the Anchor of Europe, and the Hope of the World to cherish in her bosom lawless receptacles into which the malignity, caprice, or avarice of a relation could hurry another to live in torture, and die in despair, without a hand to succour or save. But I will not reproach the laws; these evils are now made known, and will, no doubt, be remedied. Pardon, reader, this natural ebullition upon again entering on a subject I fondly hoped would never call forth the labours of my pen any more.

Upon the case of Mrs. Ellis I will make no further comments. Poor Poll, as she was called, will demand a sigh, when her persecutors are forgotten, or only remembered for their infamy.

> For in life's path though thorns abundant grow,
> Still there were joys Poor Poll could never know;
> Joys which the gay companions of her prime,
> Sipp'd as they floated on the stream of time.

LITTLE EMMA

In this nursery of vice, and shield of crime, surrounded by all the horrors that can appal mature age, and render a juvenile mind distracted, was confined a child about nine years old, who went by the name of 'Little Emma;' but it mattered not to her what she was called, for she was in a dreadful state of insanity, and it was always necessary to keep a straight-waistcoat upon her. It did not appear to me that she could articulate distinctly, but uttered gutteral sounds, such as the Hottentots at the Cape of Good Hope use. She was much neglected. Below the waistcoat, which reached her loins, she had seldom any covering whatever, and often no shoes on her feet, and her little thighs were excoriated as if by stripes; her manner was very wayward, and the keeperess used to beat her into the garden with a bamboo cane; and I once saw her seize the child by the back part of the straight waistcoat, and dash her head against the back steps, the same whereon Miss Rolleston was abused. The child seemed (I regret to say) strong and vigorous, and likely to endure its mental and body miseries for a length of time. The story I was told of this child was this: Two raving maniacs, male and female, were confined to one room in the cellar, and this was the offspring of their embraces.

I cannot vouch for the truth of this, but all the keepers and keeperesses, and even Jemmy Davis, the veteran scoundrel of Whitmore House, agreed in the same tale. I am perfectly aware that insanity is hereditary, but I am not so much versed in Gall, Spurzheim, or Lawrence,[1] to judge whether raving madness could thus be communicated from the parents to the child, nor whether it be possible for raving maniacs to procreate children; but this I know, that the horrid treatment this child experienced was such, that Warburton, his housekeeper,

---

1   Franz Josef Gall (1758 – 1828) was a German neuroanatomist, physiologist, and the founder of phrenology, a discipline subsequently popularised by physician and disciple, Johann Gaspar Spurzheim (1776 – 1832); and Sir William Lawrence, 1st Baronet FRCS FRS (1783 – 1867), a surgeon, thought mental processes were a function of the brain. —Ed.

and keeperesses, merit the severest punishment upon earth; and had I the power, the portals of heaven should be barred against their entrance, for their cruelty to the baby who never could offend, because it never had a gleam of reason to know its right hand from its left.

I feel sorry I cannot recollect the name of the brutal keeperess placed over this little maniac. She was very tall and slender, and had a visage not unlike that of the mermaid lately exhibited in St. James's Street, and she possessed about the same feeling. She was a common, or rather an uncommon strumpet, for I believe she cohabited with more than a dozen men.

MR. BLAGROVE

This gentleman is the son and heir of a very rich West India planter, and was bred to the profession of the law; when at Jamaica he caught a brain fever, from the effects of which he will not recover whilst he remains at Whitmore House. He is quite inoffensive, and not ill-treated—continually; a cut with a whip, or a knock-down blow, when he is clamorous to have his snuff box filled, is all that falls to his share; and herein I account him fortunate. He lives in the front parlour, and his father pays liberally for his board; nevertheless he is seldom decently clad; and I remember once, when his father took him out to dine and spend the day, he, as instructed, spoke in his mad way of the kindness he experienced from Davis and another, to whom Mr. Blagrove gave a guinea each; notwithstanding this, when he returned in the evening those very fellows hurried him into the porter's lodge, and robbed him of a guinea, This vile conduct was mentioned to Warburton, who said he had nothing to do with it; thus are these dens the very focus of robbery of the very worst description. To rob the dead is accounted most horrible; is it not worse to rob the living, who are dead to every feeling but those of smell and taste, and deprive the poor wretched darkened being of the only gratification he can feel-his snuff, pipes, and tobacco? I have seen the hapless creatures, after being bereft of these articles, or the price to buy them, wandering about pining with melancholy, and when any friendly hand has offered them a supply, the look they gave was so expressive, that it almost seemed the returning dawn of reason lighting up the woe worn countenance once more with the sensible glow of gratitude.

I will now for a moment pause, and ask Mr. Warburton if I have erred in a single particle of all that has preceded. I should be glad to have it in my power to contradict any part of my statements, and turn them in his favour. I am not the herald of oppression, delighting to find out things degrading to human nature; I am the advocate of suffering innocence, and wish to exalt my species. I wish not to probe a man's heart, to find it festering with corruption, but to discover it pure and uncontamminated. I am not accustomed to look upon the dark side of the picture of human life, painted by Satan, but turn to the bright, traced by the finger of Providence, where all is smiling around. I even look with friendly compassion on Mr. Warburton, and would be most happy to discover some redeeming good qualities in his heart, which I might place to the account as a set-off against all the bad I have been compelled to relate.

My feelings have been sadly lacerated in making the details of the horrid dungeon, (Whitmore House) and when I look back upon what I have done, I wonder where I got the courage to go through with it. I am still in the midst of my labour, and will persevere till I finish my duty to God and my country. It is not the atrocities of Whitmore House alone that I am able to expose, I can follow Mr. Warburton wherever he practices mad-house keeping. I have a clue to wind through all his intricacies, even though they were more puzzling than the Cretan labyrinth; and for the sake of producing facts corroborative of what I have already stated, to shew that it is not one private mad-house alone, but the whole that are bad and infamous. I will beg the reader to accompany me to the White House, Bethnal Green.

The White House,
Bethnal Green

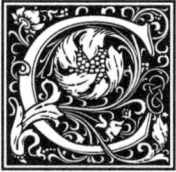

ommonly called Talbot's, but, in fact, solely Mr. Warburton's property; there he will also find I am able, as I told him before, 'to tickle his catastrophe,' and, with the blessing of God, call the sinner to repentance; if not the repentance of sincerity, that of shame and vexation, at being exposed and confounded in his operations upon human feeling.

The first case which I shall begin with, for the benefit of public information, and private gratification of Warburton, Talbot, Dunston and Co., is that of

CAPTAIN E. W. PIERCE,

A gentleman by profession, birth, education, and conduct, who suffered a martyrdom, under the care of Warburton's agents.

I recollect reading, in the Roman history, of some prisoner in a dungeon, whom his keepers, out of their tender mercy, could not kill at once, but kept him night and day awake, by pricking his flesh with their spears till he expired from exhaustion. The keepers in private mad-houses seem to be descendents of these ignoble Romans, for they keep a man constantly awake to his misery, and torture him till he dies heart-broken. This sort of torture was tried upon Captain Pierce, but the stamina of his constitution and mind defied their efforts, and his life was saved to serve as a means of exposing his persecutors.

Captain Pierce was a man of some property, which his brother wished to get possession of. It is probable that Captain Pierce was a free-liver, and rather eccentric, as most liberal minded men are, which was taken advantage of by his unnatural brother, who readily got a certificate of his insanity in the usual way, from a medical man that had never seen him, and had him seized in the street by two fellows, who forced him into a hackney-coach, and plunged him into the White House, on Bethnal Green. This kidnapping occurred on the 2nd of May, 1815, a day which will be remembered by the unsuspecting victim with emotions of horror, till the flood-gates of life are closed in everlasting rest.

Can any thing be imagined more dreadful than this; a person in his senses, following his daily vocations quietly in the street, is at once torn from liberty and light, and immured in the cells of a private mad-house. Had he been conveyed into Newgate amongst felons, there he would have hope; that is a public prison, 'open to all, and influenced by none,' his plaints would have been heard by the public authorities, and at some time he was sure of redress; but in a private mad-house, if you have a thousand friends, they are debarred from seeing you; a single relation, aided by a corrupt physician, runs you down by human blood-hounds, and at once shuts you up, treats you as a maniac, and deprives you of liberty, property, and, in time, your senses. The book of nature is closed upon you, and you only see the sky once a week, or month, as the caprice of a vulgar and inhuman keeper pleases. Brooks may murmur—trees put forth their green leaves—flowers of every hue bloom—birds sing—nature laugh on every side—and beauty smile; this you know, and the thought that you can never enjoy them, is horrible to a man of sense and understanding; and such was Captain Pierce when he was seized upon and incarcerated in the White House. There he was deprived of the use of pen and ink, daily insulted, fed ill, and badly lodged. It is of no use going into the minute particulars of his case, as no one at Whitmore House was worse treated than at the White

House, where the same cruel, uniform routine of interested villainy was practised, and, perhaps, to more perfection, as the chief, Warburton, did not visit it so often, considering it as an inferior establishment; and Talbot, the master, was well trained to 'do his duty in that state of life,' into which it had pleased Warburton to call him.

On the 12th of May, 1816, Captain Pierce was released, having been a whole twelvemonth treated as a madman, and every thing but murdered.

This case, I am told, has been before the public, as I have now, on my little table, a letter, dated the 12th of May, 1823, at Holmes's Hotel, from Captain Pierce, and addressed to me, in which he says, 'On the recovery of my liberty, I published 300 pamphlets in the form of a letter, addressed to a noble lord, stating how I had been treated.' I have never seen the pamphlet, nor has Captain Pierce one in his possession, or I should have it; however, I do not want it, and I am not sure, if I am author for using it in so good a cause; and I mention it, to let Mr. Warburton see there are more in the world than myself, ready to denounce the atrocities of his Houses. I can safely appeal to the above gentleman for the truth of my observation as to himself, but I am not indebted to him for any information on the subject whatever.

MR. COMPTON

Is the son of Doctor Compton, of Islington, and one of the King's Chaplains; he is subject to fits, or what is more commonly termed the falling sickness, a disease, often brought on, and always encreased by the use of spirituous liquors; with the knowledge of this, he is encouraged in his propensities for drinking. I mean not to hide a fact for or against the house, or any confined therein. This young man is, I am sorry to say, addicted to inebriety, but if that were a reason for confining a man, then might half London be taken up, and made subjects for Warburton's honourable care.

Mr. Compton is perfectly sane, and being well supplied with money, the keepers take care he shall never want liquors, especially when any one visits him, in order that intoxication may be mistaken for idiotic lunacy. For some time he has been more regular and reflective, and anxious to quit his den, and, in consequence, all his friends have been denied access to him; and it is a rule of private mad-houses, that no one has a right to see a patient but those who put him in; thus, where a man is confined by an interested relative, he may have many friends who are quite ignorant of his wretched situation.

Mr. Compton is very ill used, and has often been chastised for presuming to complain.

This case is a proof that these houses will receive a man under any excuse, and call it insanity. If people are to be confined for drunkenness of the brain, with impunity, in a private mad-house, I doubt not but Mr. Warburton's impudent sophistry would assert, that as passion is a drunkenness

of the mind, it must be insanity also, and stand in
need of his heavy sheltering hand.

ATROCIOUS CASES OF VIOLATION, BY PETER PARKER, OF THREE INSANE FEMALES

Ah, me! the laurel wreath that murder wears,
Blood nurs'd, and water'd by the widow's tears,
Seems not so foul, so tainted, and so dread.

If the case of Miss Rolleston was so atrocious that
it almost makes me shudder when I think upon it,
that which I am going to relate is one that exceeds
it, as much as the blackness of the Ethiop does the
whiteness of the European.

The mind may heap horror upon horrors, and
imagination descend to the depths of hell, yet there
it will find 'fiends less foul' than these employed in
private mad-houses, to torture and pollute unconscious innocence.

This monster, Peter Parker, is the house-carpen-
ter, and occasionally assists as a keeper; his office
of carpenter, at various times, gives him access to
every part of this 'prison-house,' amongst his broth-
ers in iniquity, who, no doubt, are equally guilty, but
less known. He is a sort of 'Lothario,' a braggart who
boasts of his triumphs over helpless women, whom
I should deem it worse than death to look upon with
any eyes but those of pity, and think it sacrilege to
touch, but with a protecting hand.

Men's minds are made up of strange materials, but this fellow's of the worst kind I ever heard of; no one that knows him can relate a single trait of common honesty in his character, and he is so hardened, that I may, with truth, put into his mouth the words of Aaron, the Moor, from the play of *Titus Andronicus*.

> If one good deed I ever did in all my life,
> I do repent it from my very soul.

After the many instances of horror on which we have so largely expatiated, we forbear entering into a long detail of circumstances, not wishing to shock the ear more than we can conscientiously avoid.

ANNE BALDWIN

Was a patient of a very tender age, and had she been in her perfect health and senses, quite incapable of resisting the brutal assaults of such a fellow as Parker, but she had not a spark of reason at any time to direct her ways, and was, no doubt, a passive victim in the villain's hands. She became pregnant, and brought forth a child of misery, destined never to be recognized by its mother, and if it lives, must abhor its father. What an idea must the reader have of the moral feelings and virtues of the rulers over this house of mourning and despair, when he is told, that after this deed, for which the tongue has not a name, and for which the perpetrator deserved to be instantly shot; he was suffered to remain in the house as usual, and, perhaps, continues at this day, to have access to the victim of his pollution.

MARTHA JONES

Was another wretched maniac, whose person he polluted, and she also bore a child to him. A girl, named Ellen, came within reach of his brutal lust, and, with others, whom it were useless to name, had children by him, and he is still where he was, honoured and caressed by his infernal masters.

Now, reader, let me beg your serious attention to a very few observations: I do not pretend to be a better, or wiser being than you are, but I am confident I know more of the subject on which I am writing. Is it proper that such places ought to exist in a land of liberty, or in any land on the face of the earth? The crimes of this Parker are dreadful, but they are not solitary, they are common in all private mad-houses, and I have heard instances on the truth, of which I have not a shadow of doubt, which are even worse than this. It is not in the power of man to imagine a more detestable or distressing case than that of the females thus subjected to Parker's lust, and God forbid they should ever be restored to their senses, to know what they have endured; it would be to them as a resurrection from the tomb, to endure the torments of the damned; they had better 'sleep the sleep that knows no waking;' be alive in heart-but dead in mind.

Infamous as Parker must appear to all eyes, he has still superiors and accomplices in crime, who are worse than himself—I mean those under whom he lives; his masters. Be they Warburton, Talbot, or who they may, they are seventy and seven times worse than their attendant demon; they not only permit him to proceed in his work of destruction, but they stand by and smile upon the havock he is making of nature's loveliest forms. The act of God that paralyzed the heavenly mind, excites no pity or compassion in their hearts, but added to that, they allow their servant to perpetrate the ruin of the body. They retain him in their service; he becomes endeared to them by his vices, and more useful by his capability of being base: he is, no doubt, a vile ignorant knave, born in the lowest wretchedness, and nursed on the lap of blasphemy, with intellects not superior to a brute, and no education but his masters. The Warburton's, and others, affect to be men of superior intellects and enlightened minds, into whose power are placed the sons and daughters of the first families in England, and on them be the chief blame, and on them the chief guilt. If there are any having relatives in these dreadful abodes who may read these transactions, they must feel miserable to reflect on the sorrows their misplaced confidence has inflicted upon those they held dear; and if the law awards no punishment for such crimes, I, at all events, will punish them by exposure, which may keep other victims from their racks, chains, and tortures, whereon the body is mutilated, after the vital spark is shrouded in darkness.

I promised to state worse cases than that of Miss Rolleston, and I think I have redeemed my pledge. She had a father, rolling in affluence, and basking in the sunshine of the Treasury, who was in the habit of visiting her often, yet wealth, consequence, and attention, could not save his daughter from horrible prostitution. What wonder then that such poor creatures as those I have just spoken of fell under the spoiler's dominion, and how many such have fallen, who are unknown, God only can tell. The difference in rank and fortune makes no difference in the suffering, virtue is alike the companion of those who value her company in the cottage or the palace, and I sympathize as much in the sorrows of Anne Baldwin, as in those of Miss Rolleston, and both call aloud for redress.

I have seen an able written pamphlet by Dr. Rogers, with whom I had some slight acquaintance, and have seen at Whitmore House; it is published against Warburton and his houses. This I did not know till yesterday, when the work was put into my hands'; and I am happy to find it bears me out in the truth of all my assertions, and carries the charges still higher than I have done. I give an extract from it, to shew how accordant his opinion and knowledge is with my own.

I come now to a part of my subject which more, perhaps, than even any of the facts I have already stated, will fill the reader's mind with horror and indignation.

It is not an uncommon case for female patients, married and unmarried, to become pregnant by the infernal ruffians, masters and keepers, who have the care of them, against whose designs the feeble barriers of separation, and female keepers, afford no protection. What, on recovery, must be the mental torture of a virtuous woman, the victim of these monsters, at such a retrospect? the pen drops from my hand when I think on the maddening sensations of her father—her husband.

With this I shall conclude my remarks on the cases of these unfortunate females, and leave the reader to reflect upon them—if he can; my reflection is swallowed up by indignation.

MR. ALDERTON, CHEESEMONGER, WHITECHAPEL

This is one of those lamentable cases that often occur where the patient is incapable of resisting or complaining of the barbarous usage he receives. A fellow named James Hatfield had charge of him, and for some slight cause, so pushed and knocked poor Alderton about, that he absolutely broke the wrist of his left arm. Doctor Reed observing that his arm appeared lame, enquired from what cause it arose, and the inhuman scoundrel, Hatfield, replied, that it was owing to a paralytic affection; thus depriving the poor man of every hope of assistance, and, no doubt, of the use of his arm for ever. Mr. Alderton was a man of property, upwards of sixty years of age, so that grey hairs are no protection from the assaults of these destroyers of the human race. This fellow never received even the slightest reprimand for what he had done, and is still there, sanctioned to commit more and greater crimes, whenever the barbarity of his temper excites him to do so. This fellow would, no doubt, ground his defence, if he had to make any, for committing the barbarous deed, by attributing it to accident.

I once saw Jemmy Davis—(I wish I could give this monster the damning immortality Fielding has given to Jonathan Wild, and also the same reward—a gibbet); but to the fact. I once saw Davis order a poor old patient to put his hand on his toe, whilst he drew off his boot, in doing so Davis swore at him for hurting his foot, and deliberately taking up the boot-jack, struck him on the head and knocked him down, the blood gushing out in streams; the housekeeper was passing by at the time, and I pointed out to her the brute's conduct; she questioned him, and his answer was, 'Lord love you, ma'am, I was lifting up the boot-jack, and he run his head against it by accident.' This impudent lie made me remonstrate more strongly with Mrs. Bruning when we got into the parlour, and she very humanely said, 'Ah, we must'nt notice trifles; and keepers must shew their authority now and then, or the patients would get the better of them.'

Grant me patience, kind heaven, to get to the end of this painful narrative, for every page I turn over reminds me of some fresh atrocity worthy of execration.

This Davis had a method of what he elegantly called man-handling his victims, by putting his two thumbs into their mouths, outside of their teeth, shaking their heads furiously, and often striking them against the wainscotting, or the wall. This too, I presume, he would call accident. Yes! it is accident puts people into private mad-houses-and it is by accident they are there tortured, and die. This, I have no doubt, would be Warburton's tale, if any one would credit him. There is only one real accident that ever occurs in a private mad-house, that is, when a person gets out of it alive, whose interest it is for the master to keep or kill; and that must be entirely by accident.

MR. ARCHIBALD PARK

Has been confined in the White House, under the care of Warburton's *locum tenens*, Talbot, about two years. I omitted to say that the more immediate regulation of this prison is confined to one Jennings, he is the acting manager, and 'take him for all and all,' we may say, as Jack Ketch said of his predecessor, 'He was a very nice man, and executed his business as much like a gentleman as could be expected;' so Jennings is far superior to his fellows, but still far beneath human nature.

Mr. Park was given to intoxication; and Dr. Jones of Finsbury Square, signed a certificate of his insanity; he was first sent to Whitmore House, and then removed. He suspected Dunston, the Master of Saint Luke's Hospital, of an improper intimacy with his wife; true or false, I presume not to say. He made several attempts to escape; and on his detection, had handcuffs of four pounds weight put upon his wrists, and was strapped down in bed. The horrors of these places may be conceived, when a man in this situation would think of attempting to regain his liberty. But Mr. Park did so: he contrived to slip his manacles over his hands, and actually wrenched one of the iron bars from the window, when he was discovered, and dreadfully beaten.

Bowdler the head keeper is particularly severe on Park, and is a perfect rascal.

This is one, out of the numerous cases where wives confine their husbands from improper motives. There is no doubt but Mr. Park had acted imprudently; and I am much inclined to believe what I have heard respecting her and Dunston, from the circumstance of her totally neglecting and abandoning him to the mercy of monsters.

DR. WILLIAMS, OF WANTAGE, BERKS

This much oppressed man is well known and highly respected at Wantage. His daughter eloped from her parental home, which had the effect of rendering him melancholy. His wife went to Oxford, and upon her representations, Dr. Watt, a convenient physician, signed a certificate of her husband's insanity, whom he had not seen on the occasion; and on that authority was Dr. Williams put into the White House, where I apprehend he will terminate his miserable existence.

The keepers laugh at his complaints, which are very few, for the lash is ready for all who dare to hint even a wish to be out side of the walls. It never happens that these fellows report the recovery of any one of their friends, unless those friends are in the habit of visiting the patient, and watching his progress, they then make a merit of necessity, and at the same time they state that if the patient is sufficiently well to be taken away, they always advise his friends to let him remain a little longer, for fear of a relapse; thus clinging to the last shilling that can be extracted, under pretence of tenderness and care, when, in fact, it is out raging humanity.

Amongst the many sufferers confined in these disgraceful places, are a considerable number of naval and military officers, whose openness of character has been taken advantage of by interested relatives. Amongst the former profession

CAPTAIN WILLIAM FORBES LEITH

Has suffered severely. A love attachment was the cause. He had paid his addresses to a lady of family and fortune; but as Captain Leith, though of a family ancient as her own, had only his pay to support him in the rank of a gentleman; the lady's friends discountenanced his attentions, and removed her to different places to prevent their meeting. He, with the true spirit of a British seaman, kept up the chace; so fair a prize was not to be given up by any obstacles, however dangerous. But what open hostilly could not effect, was done by stratagem.

Captain Leith, it seems, had no relations in England who appeared to care for him. The lady's friends procured a testimony of the Captain's insanity from a country physician; had him seized at a distance from London, and hurried up to the White House—distance is nothing to Warburton; he sends his myrmidons to the most distant parts of the kingdom. This is a proper place to remark, that whenever a letter comes to him from a family who suspect any of its members to be affected with insanity, and suppose that a keeper from Warburton's will satisfy their doubts; and if painfully true, do the unfortunate person good; before the keeper goes, Warburton puts a certificate into his pocket, signed by a London physician, who cannot have seen the person, and gives him strong injunctions, FIRST, to persuade the family that the person is insane. SECONDLY, that he will be cured if sent to Whitmore House. I have known Warburton to do this twenty times, but I am wearied of relating such acts of rascallity.

In the White House Captain Leith remonstrated in vain; he might as well have whistled to the wind;

and to add to the horrors of his confinement, he was treated as an insane person, and by day and night always kept with the maniacs.

He managed, at last, to have some communication with his riends, and they opened a correspondence with the family which confined him—an understanding took place—an arrangement was made—in which Captain Leith sacrificed his own feelings to those of the object of his regard, and he once more came forth to breathe a pure air, with an impaired constitution, which has compelled him to go to the South of France, doubtful if he ever may return. He has not prosecuted Warburton for the reasons above mentioned, and I am very sorry that through his tenderness and generosity of heart the guilty have, for the present, escaped punishment.

This case shews that no man is safe from the reach of mad-house keepers. It was strangers who had Captain Leith arrested—and strangers that detained him. At this rate, any one that bears another enmity, has only to apply to a private mad-house, and get him seized and imprisoned for life—for it may be seen by nearly all the preceding cases, that the medical men make no scruple to sign their name to a man's lunacy, upon the *ip se dixit* of such an interested being as Warburton. I have often seen Tom Harris, Warburton's head confidential keeper, sent to get a certificate of insanity signed by a physician, with merely the name of the person written on a slip of paper, with orders if he could not find one physician, to go to another—and another still—till it was done; for he had a regular set in pay, ready to do his bidding.

After having perused the above oppressive case, my reader, who may be in pursuit of some fair object, whose connections are adverse to his views, will keep a sharp look out; for instead of being 'called out' for his presumption, to give honourable satisfaction, he stands a chance of being taken up by the private mad-house bloodhounds, to gratify dishonourable revenge.

What a distressing case is this of Captain Leith, a brave officer who has been shedding his best blood in defence of the liberties of his country, returns into her bosom—into the realms his valour had saved, to partake of those liberties he so dearly won—but is instantly seized upon and made a slave: he hopes to enjoy a tranquil evening after a long and stormy day, but all his hopes are blighted in the bud—he is immured in a dungeon, though guiltless of crime; and, instead of the thunder of cannon he so often pointed for Britain's sake, the yellings of maniacs din his ears, and he is condemned to the society of madmen—and for what? because there are people so mean as to seek revenge by base means; and private mad-house keepers ready to aid and abet their nefarious schemes. But I trust I am giving the death-blow to those infernal inquisitions

> Which hold alike the coward and the brave,
> Where every freeman is a wretched slave.

MR. JOHNSON,

Whose case I mentioned in page 30 of Part First, is now wandering about like a weary pilgrim, over a path covered with briars and thorns, in search of a green sod to lay his head upon, and die; but which he is destined never to find. He has passed twenty-six years of his miserable existence in these horrible Bastilles, without ever going beyond the walls, except on his removal from one prison to another, and once when he attempted to escape. I could almost persuade myself that God would permit suicide in such a case, and pardon the unhappy man for flying from such horrible prospects into his presence a few years before his appointed time.

Mr. Johnson is an American by birth; and fought on the side of Great Britain, for which she permitted him to spend his days in one of her private gaols. He had some property-I think he told me seven hundred a-year-which laid in America; he came to England to prosecute a claim relative to losses during the war, when his relations followed—threw him into a private mad house, and seized upon all he had!

A liberal allowance, however, was allotted for his support; and he was decently taken care of till the death of his friends, when Warburton, as he always does on these occasions, asserted, that they had left scarce sufficient to support him; and for that reason removed him to the White House.

His keepers—or the keepers, for he wanted none—who had known him for many years, told me he had never been more insane than he was at the moment I saw him, when he was perfectly composed.

He appears resigned to his fate; and looks forward to peace, where his tyrants may look with despair, in

Another and a better world.

I could multiply without end the cases of distress in this house, but the reader must be tired, as well as myself, with a constant repetition of enormities over which the eye glances with a tremulous motion; and the heart throbs with the most painful anxiety.

Mr. Talbot has just about as much feeling as his friend, Warburton. Vulgar, rude, boisterous, and forbidding; he has none of the outward signs of any inward grace; and like his great master, has been exposed, more than once, in open court. That he is an ungrateful fellow, and a false friend, is very evident, from the trial, 'DENNIS *versus* TALBOT;' when it appeared, he was the friend and companion of Mr. Dennis, but for reasons best known to himself, he joined in a plan with his half uncle, to have him arrested; placed two ruffians in the young man's house, and held a jury on him, of which that worthy man, Warburton, was foreman. By the firmness of a friend, all these invaders were driven out, and Mr. Dennis restored to liberty. Rogues are always cowards: and Talbot took care to be out of the way. The trial is worthy of a reading, just to appreciate properly Mr. Talbot's brutish qualities. The damages given were £300 —it ought to have been £3000. Mr. Warburton cares little for such a sum, in supporting any of his myrmidons, and what he calls the reputation of his houses-what reputation they bear since I have thrown them open to public view, is such that no private house could stand by it.

ON THE INTERNAL ARRANGEMENTS IN THE WHITE HOUSE

Whitmore House is a spacious building, with good gardens; and in every respect well calculated for the purposes of a private receptacle for lunatics. I have said so much of it in the course of this Work, that I decline further remarks; but will say a few words of the White House. It is quite inconvenient; and a small yard, twenty-three yards long, by twenty yards wide, is the only place where One Hundred and Fifty patients can take air and exercise! It is surrounded by a wall sixteen feet high! It is a perfect sink, where you breathe pestilence, and tread in pollution. The patients have malt liquor *ad libitum*, and spirits are brought in, by the keepers, to all who have money; and whom they compel to treat them. Thus every afternoon drunkenness is the order of the day. A lamentable instance of this baneful indulgence is found in a person named Chisscomb; he was recovering very fast, but, unfortunately, his friends sent him a supply of money, when he was encouraged to drink so enormously of spirits, that he went raving mad, and was sent to Saint Luke's.

The keepers are more frequently drunk here, than at Whitmore House. Fisher, a brute, who had sixty unfortunate human beings under his care, was one day so drunk, that a patient, Captain Price, of the Royal Navy, (nearly related to Archdeacon Price) had to lead him to his bed; realizing the fable of the 'Lambs protecting the Wolves.' This Fisher was the only instance I remember of one of these fellows being punished, after a long intimacy with the intrigues of the house; but self-interest prompted them to do it. He was sent out one night, to take care of a celebrated composer of music, (Mr. Ireland) and got so drunk as to be incapable of doing his duty, and was dismissed; his unfeeling conduct to his patients was never noticed, but when once his employers were touched, he was punished.

It is customary in this house also, to let the keepers have the patients' old clothes, as perquisites, which they sold to the master, who supplied them to the parish patients, charging them as new.

Miss Ford is also aware of the abuses in the linen-room; and the keepers often make the patients say they are sick, in order that medicine may be given them, and they accumulate empty phials to sell to the Jews.

I advance nothing but what I am ready and willing to testify upon oath, or to prove it at the Bar of the House of Commons, (if required) and defy the ingenuity of Warburton to find out a place where I am incorrect.

I shall conclude these statements with a very brief account of what is not generally known:—

DISMISSAL OF JAMES DAVIS FROM WINDSOR, FOR KICKING AND STRIKING HIS LATE MAJESTY, KING GEORGE THE THIRD,

The keepers in attendance on his late Majesty at Windsor, were, by the recommendation of Doctor Willis, sent from Whitmore House. Mr. Warburton selected for the purpose a relation of his, named Penlington, who formerly kept a little huckster's-shop; he was a notorious drunkard, very vulgar, mean in manners, in mind, and in form. The only good qualification he possessed, was a knack at telling truth, for which reason I doubted his relationship to Warburton very much. Another of them had been a journeyman baker at Bristol; and a third was a bricklayer's labourer; a fourth, a man whose name must be ringing in the ears of all who have read this work, famous for every quality that can disgrace a man—Jemmy Davis; these were the precious fellows employed about the person of a helpless, blind, and good old King. Fellows whose touch would taint putridity itself, and render it more abominable. These fellows were appointed to attend to his comforts, and handle his august person whenever necessity demanded it; though I have no doubt but they were called 'gentlemen' by Warburton. There is an old saying, 'Jack is as good as his Master,' in this case it was true.

There were always some rays of reason, emanating by faint flashes, at distant intervals, from the King, like sparks from a dying taper, placed in a drear and dark apartment. He knew the men by the sound of their voices, and would feel with his fingers, if the King's arms were stamped on the covers of the bibles he made them carry; he found, once, that it was not the case, and was much irritated; what a lesson this for human pride. Upon a certain occasion, it became necessary to use a straight waistcoat. Davis was as strong as he was brutal.

> Oh it is excellent to have a giant's strength; but
> tyrannous to use it like a giant!
> —SHAKESPEARE.

The other keepers strove by gentle means to quiet their Royal Patient; but Davis, who imagined himself handling some poor wretch at Whitmore House, struck his Majesty a severe blow betwixt his shoulders, then pulling with all his force at the strings, he shook his body backwards and forwards, and kicked him repeatedly behind, till the unfortunate Monarch screamed with pain. Penlington drove him away, and the circumstances made such an impression on the King, that he was dreadfully ill for many days, more from a wounded spirit than a wounded frame, for he was keenly sensible of indignity, and never forgot who he was; he often muttered about this event, and it left a lasting painful impression on his mind, till every impression was lost in torpor. Whenever he saw Davis, his Majesty revolted at his sight, shuddered, and exclaimed, as he did at Warburton's long nose, 'Take him away, take him away;' and at last, Davis was dismissed, but only to Whitmore House, where he afterwards practised all those enormities I have laid to his charge. If any one had a doubt of the dreadful deeds of this miscreant, they will be dispelled when they find him, thus unable to repress his brutal disposition, and exercising his vengeance on the sacred person of the Monarch of England.

Mr. Warburton affects to be a very loyal man, and is a member of the Pitt Club, wearing a medal at his breast as large as a pewter plate; yet, instead of punishing Davis for this brutal outrage on the person of the King, he rewarded him, by giving him charge over a hundred patients, and making him second keeper at Whitmore House. Shame on such loyalty! say I.

On Private Mad-Houses
in General

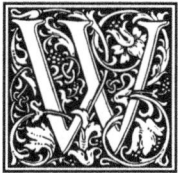

We did purpose to have offered an elaborate opinion on improvements which might be made in the nature of private mad-houses, but on a careful retrospect of our work, we think the impartial reader will agree with us, that they ought not to exist under any modification, but be abolished for ever; in this, many men of talent agree with us, who speak from serious reflection, and painful experience.

To punish what has either been arbitrarily ordered, or tacitly permitted, as far as it is possible to do so, is certainly a good object; but a far greater consideration is to prevent the practicability of the recurrence of such evils.

All the art of man will not prevent tyranny, fraud, and debauchery, from being exercised in any private establishment, the property of one interested individual, and in which, from one to three hundred of both sexes are confined, whether in or out of their senses.

The principles upon which private mad-houses stand, are hostile to the free spirit of the British constitution. I believe I called them before lawless houses, under the sanction of the law, for they are licensed. With reference to our 'prison laws,' they form an *imperium et imperio,* and with all and more power than the public prisons, they are subject to no public controul, and obey no public code of general discipline, impartially exercised for the good of all confined. They are not liable to be visited by Magistrates, Members of Parliament, or Juries; the master cannot be called to account for the authority he exercises therein, for it is his private house, where he locks up the King's subjects in defiance of the King, or rather of those laws the King is bound to see administered, for the good of all, from the highest to the lowest, who live under his sway.

The keepers are under no political or moral restraint, but each of them 'doeth that which seemeth right in his own eyes;' within the walls their will is the law, and injustice is their will; or, as Jack Cade said, so say these keepers, 'burn all the records, henceforth my mouth shall be the Parliament of England;' and so it is within the black sphere of their jurisdiction.

These houses also have raised up a set of men, who exercise a power more despotic than that of a Mahometan Cadi, and yet no law acknowledges them, and every law condemns them. No man can be condemned without the judgment of his Peers; to this wholesome fact the conduct of these men everyday gives the lie, for they condemn and imprison for life, on the authority of their own single opinion; I mean the physicians, who, by signing a certificate, whether true or false, can throw into a secret dungeon any free-born Englishman now walking the streets of London.

An Englishman's house is no longer his boasted castle. By virtue of an order from a bribed physician, (as he receives a fee for every *Lettre de Cachet* he signs) my door is liable to be entered by ruffians, upon the same principle as general warrants formerly were issued, and I can be dragged from my bed, and locked up from society, without hopes of even having my cause heard at a future day, before a jury of my country; whilst my property is confiscated to the uses of other men, and I am branded as a mad-man, because one rascally mad doctor says I am, and a mad-house has received my body.

I will not trouble my readers with arguing upon the illegality of these houses—it is evident they are so; admitting they are not illegal, the damning facts in this book, which are only a few out of a thousand, is sufficient to shew that an instant remedy ought to be applied; but the caustic will not eat away the sore—the wound is gangrened at the core, and widely spreading, to the injury of the body politic; it must be totally eradicated, and a new system of health established, all else is useless.

The subject is well worthy legislatorial attention. Have we no humane Member of Parliament, who would undertake the task of rescuing Englishmen from slavery? Where is Mr. Wilberforce?[1] 'Sleepest thou, or wakest thou, Lady Fair?' He can whine, and cant about black slaves, and racks, and chains, on the African coast, and yet sleep soundly on his feather-bed at home, within a stone's throw of dungeons, where his brother Britons, in the full vigour of sense and reason, are pining upon straw, and he knows it, and will not try to relieve them, because, perhaps, it would annoy his friends—the Ministers.

Establishments something on the plan of our excellently conducted and well regulated public hospitals, should be built, and males and females separated from each other; they should be open to public inspection, and no man ought to be consigned into them as a patient, until a jury of twelve of his nearest neighbours have pronounced him insane. But this is only intended as a hint. I would leave it to men of better and abler judgment than

---

1   William Wilberforce (1759 - 1833), an independent politician, led the movement to abolish the slave trade. —Ed.

myself. I have done my duty; I have pointed out the disease; it is for them to find the remedy, mine is but a 'bird's-eye view,' in an extensive champaign, where the flowers of corruption are shedding their baleful blossoms; where the poisoned Upas tree of Java stands in the centre, surrounded by a hedge of thorns and briars, thickly intertwisted with hemlock and deadly night-shade. It is time the tree was cut down, the land purified, the barrier-hedge trampled upon, and a free circulation of air admitted, to renovate all that have had the misfortune to breathe the pollutions of its dreadful enclosure.

I have now done: if any one feels offended, then he loves not his country and fellow-countrymen as he ought, and I heed not his censure or his praise; the good and the virtuous will applaud my intentions, and with that I am contented.

I can only say, that as I have been the first to expose these enormities, I also will be the first to come forward, if my country calls me, to prove that I have made no statement that has not truth for its foundation.

THE END

Index

Parker, Peter (rapist) 80, 81,
82, 83
Parliament vi, 8, 19, 102, 103,
104, 109, 110
Parnell, Sir Henry 18
Parthians 69
Penlington (relation of Warburton) 3, 97, 98
Perceval, Lady Bridget vi, vii,
27, 28, 29, 30, 38, 39
Persians 50, 69
Pierce, Captain E. W. (patient)
76, 77, 78
Pitt Club 25, 99
Pitt the Younger, William 25,
41, 99
Portsmouth, John Charles
Wallop, 3rd Earl of 1
Price, Captain (patient) 96
Prince Regent. *See* George IV
Princess of Wales. *See* Caroline
of Brunswick-Wolfenbüttel,
Princess of Wales

R

Redesdale, John Freeman-Mitford, 1st Baron v, vi, vii, 27,
30, 48
Reed, Dr 85
Richards, Mr 6, 37, 49
Rogers, John Wilson 84
Rolleston, Miss 10, 12, 13, 26,
42, 44, 71, 80, 84
Rolleston, Stephen 10, 11
Romans 76, 110
Rome 69, 110
Royal Navy 20, 96

S

Sangrado, Doctor (fictional
character) 4
Scarron, Mrs (patient) 53
Shakespeare, William 42, 63, 111
Sidmouth, Henry Addington,
1st Viscount vi, vii, 23, 24
Speaker of the House of Commons 9
Starfford, Earl of. *See* Wentworth, 1st Earl of Strafford,
Thomas
Star, The (newspaper) 38
St Giles 44
St Luke's Hospital for Lunatics
96

T

Talbot, Matthew (Superintendent of the White House,
Bethnal Green) 75, 78, 83,
87, 94, 95
Taylor, Miss (Warburton's
mistress) 3, 14, 111
The News (Sunday paper) 29
Troy vii, 42
Tullibardine, John Murray,
Marquis of 24, 41

V

Vestals 69
Vicar of Wakefield, The (Goldsmith) 2

W

Wakefield, Priscilla 25
Wantage 88

www.ingramcontent.com/pod-product-compliance
Lightning Source LLC
Chambersburg PA
CBHW020347100426
42812CB00035B/3382/J

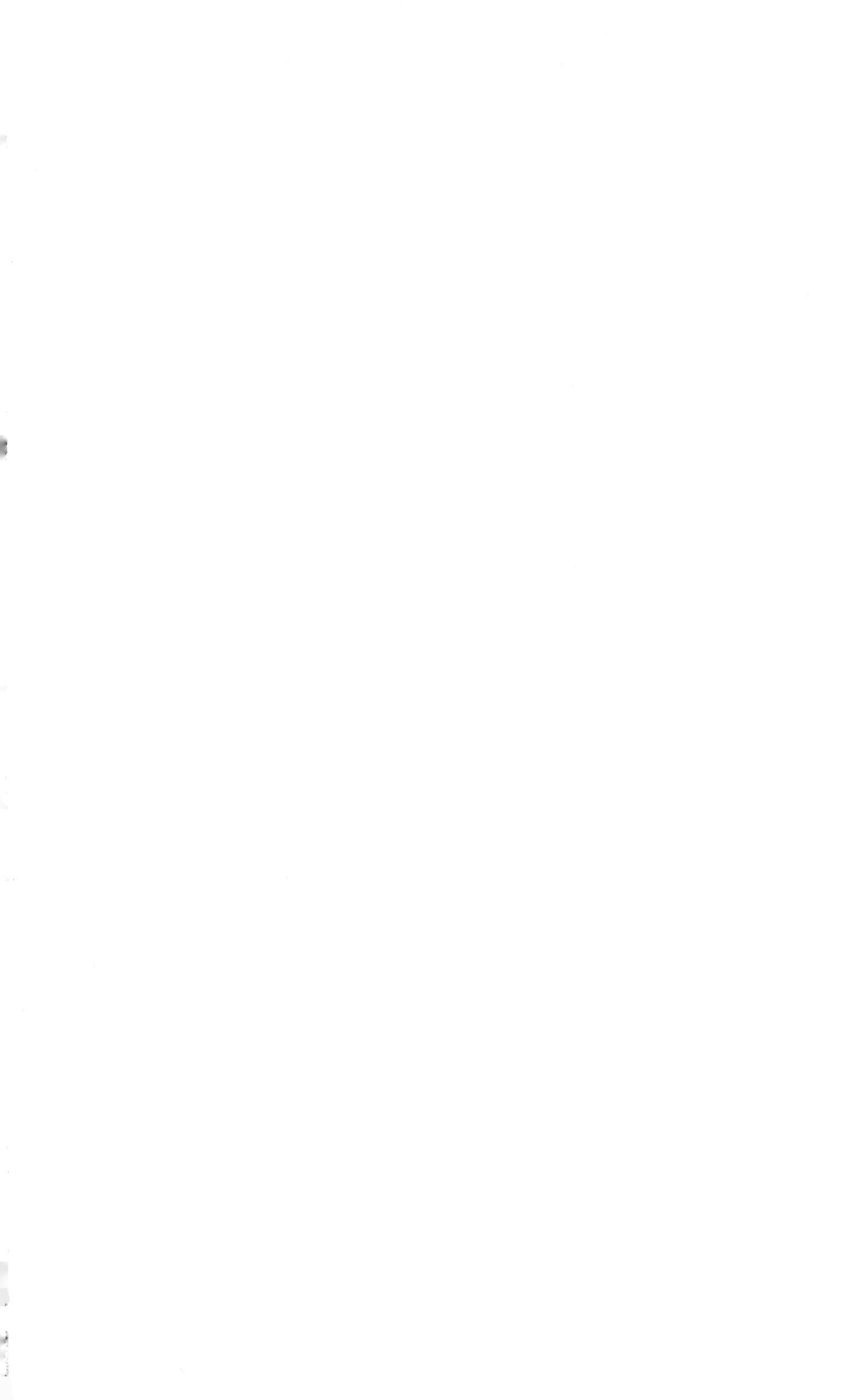